Negotiating a Good Death
Euthanasia in the Netherlands

Negotiating a Good Death
Euthanasia in the Netherlands

Robert Pool, PhD

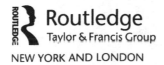

Routledge
Taylor & Francis Group

NEW YORK AND LONDON

First published 2000 by
The Haworth Press, Inc., 10 Alice Street, Binghamton, NY 13904-1580

This edition published 2013 by Routledge
711 Third Avenue, New York, NY 10017
2 Park Square, Milton Park, Abingdon, Oxon OX14 4RN

Routledge is an imprint of the Taylor & Francis Group, an informa business

Cover design by Monica L. Seifert.

Previously published in the Netherlands by WYT under the title, "Vragen om te sterven."

Library of Congress Cataloging-in-Publication Data

Pool, Robert, 1955-
    Negotiating a good death : euthanasia in the Netherlands / Robert Pool.
      p. cm.
    Includes bibliographical references and index.
    ISBN 0-7890-1080-1 (hard : alk. paper)—ISBN 0-7890-1081-X (soft : alk. paper)
    1. Assisted suicide—Netherlands. 2. Euthanasia—Netherlands. I. Title.

R726 .P66 2000
179.7—dc21
                                                       00-038286

To those who died

ABOUT THE AUTHOR

Robert Pool, PhD, studied cultural anthropology at the University of Amsterdam. He specialized in medical anthropology, receiving his doctorate in 1989. He has carried out anthropological research in India, the Netherlands, Cameroon, Tanzania, and Uganda on topics ranging from AIDS, malnutrition, and euthanasia, to sexual behavior, food taboos, and witchcraft.

Since 1996 he has been in charge of social science in the Medical Research Council (U.K.) Programme on AIDS in Uganda. Dr. Pool has published widely on medical anthropology and is the author of *Dialogue and the Interpretation of Illness: Conversations in a Cameroon Village* (1994).

CONTENTS

Preface

Euthanasia in the Netherlands: Twenty-Five Years of Debate

In spite of all the recent debates, policy shifts, and publicity, euthanasia and assisted suicide remain illegal in the Netherlands, covered by two articles in the Dutch Penal Code:

> **293:** He who takes the life of another at the latter's explicit and serious request will be punished with a prison term not exceeding twelve years or a fine in the fifth category [100,000 guilders/$50,000].

> **294:** He who purposely incites another person to suicide, assists him with suicide, or furnishes him with the means will, if suicide results, be punished with a prison term not exceeding three years.

Although the first case was tried in 1952, the broad public debate on euthanasia in the Netherlands is generally said to have started with the trial, in 1973, of a doctor who killed her terminally ill mother with an injection of morphine. The doctor was convicted of contravening Article 293 and given a one-week suspended sentence. By imposing a largely symbolic sentence, the court accepted that if a doctor's actions conformed to certain criteria, then, in practice, he or she was justified in responding to an explicit request for euthanasia.

In the ensuing years, a debate has been waged, by politicians, jurists, lobbyists, and the media, on whether euthanasia should be legalized and where the line should be drawn between acceptable and unacceptable life-terminating acts. Various pieces of draft legislation have been considered by parliament, and in the wake of election promises, commissions have been formed to investigate the possibilities and to make recommendations. However, the actual legalization of euthanasia has remained a difficult issue in the compromising postelection environment of Dutch coalition politics.

In the meantime, Dutch jurisprudence continued to develop through a series of "show trials," and although euthanasia remained illegal, rules of due care (*zorgvuldigheidsregels*) developed and became generally accepted as sufficient grounds for not prosecuting doctors who performed euthanasia. During these years, the Association for Voluntary Euthanasia played a major role in attaining broad social acceptability for the idea of voluntary euthanasia.

In the 1984 *Alkmaar* case, the Supreme Court accepted a doctor's appeal against a conviction for euthanizing a patient, claiming that a lower court had insufficiently taken into account the extent to which, according to "responsible medical opinion measured by prevailing standards of medical ethics, a situation of necessity [*noodtoestand*] had prevailed" (Enthoven 1988:94). When, as Leo Enthoven put it, the Ministry of Justice had finished with the doctor—and the doctor had finished with the Ministry of Justice—the judges had finally found a way to allow euthanasia without legalizing it: discharged from prosecution because of necessity as a result of a conflict of duties (Enthoven 1988:94).

In the same year as the *Alkmaar* decision, the Royal Dutch Medical Association published its position on euthanasia, in which it described the conditions for justifiable euthanasia.

Also in 1984 a small liberal political party, D66, submitted a proposal to parliament to legalize euthanasia by doctors if they acted in conformity with the rules of due care. Although there was wide support for this proposed legislation, the realities of coalition politics made its implementation impossible. Since then the public debate has continued as to whether euthanasia should be legalized or remain illegal, but with the possibility of avoiding prosecution through abiding by the rules of due care.

In 1985, the State Committee on Euthanasia published a report in which euthanasia was defined as the deliberate termination of a person's life by another person at the former's request. This definition gradually replaced all others and has become *the* definition of euthanasia in the public debate in the Netherlands as well as the basis for all legislation and other rules relating to euthanasia. This definition has rendered distinctions between active and passive euthanasia and between voluntary and involuntary euthanasia redundant: in the Netherlands, officially, euthanasia is, *by definition,* voluntary and active.[1]

In 1989, a new labor-Christian democratic coalition government announced the formation of the Commission of Inquiry into Medical Practice Concerning Euthanasia, popularly known as the Remmelink Commission, after its chairman. The commission was set up because of the realization that little was actually known about the nature and extent of euthanasia in practice. It was decided that the study should not be limited to euthanasia as strictly defined but include a wider range of related practices as well, referred to as "medical decisions concerning the end of life."

In 1990 to 1991, a national survey was therefore carried out by a team led by professor Paul Van der Maas to investigate the nature and incidence of euthanasia in the Netherlands, with a view to developing new legislation. To facilitate the study, the Ministry of Justice and the Royal Dutch Medical Association agreed to officially institute a notification procedure according to which doctors who carried out euthanasia would not be prosecuted if their actions conformed to the rules of due care. The results of the Remmelink study were published in 1991 (Van der Maas, Van Delden, and Pijnenborg 1991), and as a result of the study, the notification procedure was legally enacted through an amendment to the Burial Act in 1994. Because Article 293 remained unaltered, euthanasia had not been legalized, but the existing situation was now anchored in law: if doctors kept to the rules of due care and did not enter a natural cause of death on the death certificate (i.e., reported the death as euthanasia), then they would not be prosecuted.

This led some optimistic politicians to declare that the euthanasia debate in the Netherlands was now closed. In fact, the debate has continued in all its intensity, and new trials have led to further shifts in Dutch jurisprudence. In the same year that the Burial Act was amended, the Supreme Court came to a decision in the *Chabot* case, in which a psychiatrist had assisted in the suicide of a patient who was extremely depressed, but not physically ill; that is, her suffering was purely mental. Chabot had conformed to the rules of due care, though he had not actually had his patient examined by another physician, and he had notified the authorities. He was prosecuted and invoked the defense of necessity. The Supreme Court decided that there was no reason why the defense of necessity should not apply in the case of mental suffering, but that the patient should have been examined by an independent colleague. The defense of necessity failed, and Chabot was found guilty, though no penalty was imposed. Mental suffering was now seen as justifiable grounds for granting a euthanasia request.

In 1995, the ministers of justice and health commissioned a second national survey to investigate changes in practices since the Remmelink survey and to evaluate the notification procedure. This study, carried out by Professors Gerrit Van der Wal and Paul Van der Maas, concluded that end-of-life decision making had changed slightly, that no unacceptable increase in the number of such decisions had occurred, and that substantial progress had been made in the reporting and monitoring of physician-assisted death (Van der Maas et al. 1996; Van der Wal et al. 1996).

In 1997, a labor-liberal cabinet that included D66, the party that had previously proposed to legalize euthanasia, announced that euthanasia was not to be legalized in the short term, though future legalization was not excluded. In the meantime, the government proposed an adjustment to the present notification procedure, involving the establishment of multidisciplinary review commissions. This move was intended to further decriminalize (justifiable) euthanasia and thus increase the willingness of doctors to notify (Legemate and Dillman 1998:3).

At present, the rules of due care are as follows:

1. A voluntary, well-considered, and persistent request by the patient
2. Unbearable, enduring, and hopeless suffering
3. Consultation with an independent colleague
4. A written report
5. Consultation with other care providers who are involved with the patient
6. The avoidance of unnecessary suffering among relatives

7. A doctor who is present or accessible
8. The doctor's actions carried out with sufficient care (Legemate 1998:32-38)

THE PRESENT STUDY

In spite of the wealth of data generated by the Remmelink Commission survey, various aspects of the social context of euthanasia[2] remained largely opaque. To shed more light on these aspects, I carried out a two-year anthropological study (1991 to 1993), mainly among doctors, in the pulmonology, gastroenterology, AIDS, and intensive care units of a medium-sized hospital (400 beds) in the large Randstad conurbation in the western Netherlands. The study focused on how euthanasia requests develop, how doctors and nurses react to such requests, which nonmedical factors influence the decision-making process, and how this effects the reporting of euthanasia.[3]

This generated in-depth case studies of the social contexts of fifty-five deaths, in thirty of which euthanasia or related end-of-life decisions played an important role. The patients studied were selected from outpatient clinics and from the wards. They had been diagnosed as having an incurable and fatal disease (mostly cancer and AIDS) and had either already broached the topic of euthanasia or the doctor thought they were likely to raise it during the course of their illness.[4] I was in the hospital on a daily basis and present during all relevant outpatient consultations, rounds on the wards, and discussions among staff. Though not a native of the Netherlands, I had studied and worked there for fifteen years, and I had a native-speaker proficiency in Dutch. As a result, I had both a thorough understanding of the cultural context and could always understand what was being said. Most of the conversations and discussions during these activities were recorded and transcribed. In addition, all participants were interviewed frequently and in-depth, and all interviews were also recorded and transcribed. The study was explained to all participants (doctors, nurses, patients, and their relatives), and all aspects of the research were based on informed consent.

In this book, I present ten detailed case studies of euthanasia and related end-of-life decisions (Chapters 1 through 5 and 7 through

10) in which I emphasize the unique and individual nature of each case. In Chapter 11, I bring these case studies together and discuss some of the more general issues that emerged. This discussion draws on data from all the cases that I studied. Chapter 12 discusses the definition of euthanasia and the distinctions between various categories of life-terminating actions as they are used in the Netherlands. Chapter 6 is a "reflexive intermezzo" in which I present a discussion among the doctors about the drafts of my first five chapters.

The situations described in the following pages have not been altered in any way. Only the names of persons and that of the hospital have been changed, as have some of the dates, in order to protect the privacy of those involved. All conversations have been transcribed verbatim from the tapes, with only slight editing to improve readability and exclude repetition.

Robert Pool

Acknowledgments

The research on which this book is based was made possible by financial support from the Foundation for Law and Public Administration (REOB) and the Ministry of Justice in the Netherlands. In the planning phase of the study, I had fruitful discussions with Leo Enthoven, Prof. C. Van der Meer, Dr. Pieter Admiraal, Prof. E. Borst-Eilers, Prof. H. W. A. Hilhorst, Dr. D. Dos Reis Miranda, Dr. J. H. Zwaveling, Prof. F. C. B. Van Wijmen, Mr. W. Melief, Dr. G. Van der Wal, Prof. P. Van der Maas, Dr. L. Pijnenborg, and Prof. C. Spreeuwenberg.

Once the research plan had been developed, a steering committee was convened, consisting of Prof. L. C. M. Meijers, Prof. E. Borst-Eilers, Prof. H. W. A. Hilhorst, Dr. D. Dos Reis Miranda, Mr. G. J. Veerman, and Ms. A. Slotboom, who was later succeeded by Ms. M. Kockelkoren. The committee served as a forum for fruitful discussions about all aspects of the study, and I am grateful for their comments, suggestions, advice, and support. A particular word of thanks is due to Prof. Borst-Eilers for her countless suggestions and wise advice, right from the very inception of the study: her contribution was indispensable. Moreover, without her introductions to relevant people and institutions and her faith in the researcher, the study would have been impossible.

Three colleagues who became close friends during the study—Hans Werdmölder, executive secretary of REOB, and Anne-Mei The and Marijke Notermans, who carried out their own related research as part of the same project—also deserve a special word of thanks for their support in difficult moments and, after the research had been completed, for their suggestions and comments on the manuscript.

I would also like to thank Fester Possel, Chris Kruze, Jan Bakker, Tineke Pijper-Spel, and Jitske van de Akker. It is not often that the bureaucratic and administrative aspects of a research project are carried out in such an efficient and friendly manner.

In the final phase of the project, during which the report was being rewritten into a book, I profited from suggestions and advice from Cor Spreeuwenberg, Paul Van der Maas, Loes Pijnenborg, Gerrit Van der Wal, Monya Lange, Peter van Peer, and Christie Klauke.

I am most indebted, however, to the participants in the Randstad Hospital. I would like to thank the doctors, nurses, and other care providers; the director; and the patients and their relatives for their cooperation and their trust.

Chapter 1

Death and the Anthropologist:
On the Problem of Studying Euthanasia

THE END: THE DEATH OF DAVID

One Tuesday morning just before Christmas I was on my way to the AIDS ward when I ran into Dr. Edelman.

"It's all set for this morning, half past eleven," he said. He was nervous. "And I still have to arrange everything," he called over his shoulder as he rushed down the corridor, his white coat flapping behind him. He was talking about David's euthanasia. David was one of his patients.

I had seen David often during my more than one and a half years' research in the hospital—idling down the corridor in his training suit, a packet of cigarettes in his hand; talking in a friendly voice to other patients or to one of the nurses; or sitting quietly in his room absorbed in a Stephen King thriller.

David had signed a euthanasia declaration[1] more than six months previously, and one day, I asked him why he had done so.

"My partner died two years ago," he said in a quiet voice. "He held out to the very last day. He suffered—I could see he was suffering—and there's no way that I would want to go through *that*. It would be too much. So I think the good part of it is that I can say when. I'm in control. Dr. Edelman has known me for going on two years now. He knows that I'm not the type of person who would ask for something like that if I didn't mean it."

The names of all doctors, nurses, aides, patients, and relatives throughout this book have been changed to protect the subjects' identities.

Dr. Edelman's promise to accede to David's euthanasia request in due course had a safety function: it was a guarantee that he need not suffer more than he wanted to. But he didn't intend to die just yet.

"I think I've still got a couple of good months in me," he said. "The important point is that when the time comes there's somebody there who is willing to help me. . . . I think it's good to . . . to . . . set the foundations now."

The day after our talk he was discharged, and I thought I would not see him again for some time. Two days later, however, I went into the ward kitchen to pour myself some coffee and ran into David.

"You're back again," I said, surprised.

"Yes," he said. "I was admitted this morning. It didn't work out at home. I couldn't manage. I've realized that I can't live outside the hospital anymore."

"What couldn't you manage, the shopping?"

"No," he said emphatically. "That's not a problem. Somebody does that for me. It's just . . . it just didn't work. I couldn't manage alone. I've decided that I've had enough," he said.

His euthanasia request had become actual; he had decided to ask Dr. Edelman to set a date.

Later that day I asked him about the reasons for this sudden change of mind.

"Well, the thing is, I still feel pretty good, . . . " he hesitated and looked embarrassed. "I resemble something out of a . . . Steven King horror. Let me show you." He leaned back in his chair and pulled up his T-shirt. His body was bright yellow and his chest and stomach were covered with round blotches the size of large coins. They were purplish-black in the middle and lighter toward the edges, where they became a greenish halo that gradually merged with the surrounding yellow. The spots were more or less the same size and evenly spaced. His skin was hard and scaly, reptilian.

"The way I look was always very important to me." He smiled ruefully and fell silent. "I'm sure that whatever it is that's making me yellow can't be doing me any good," he went on. "It must be slowly poisoning me. I don't want to wait until the last moment and then have to beg for release." He fell silent again.

"And also," he resumed after a moment, "I believe . . . you know, about death and that sort of thing."

"What do you believe?" I asked.

"Well, I believe that we don't just . . . blink into nothingness. . . . I think there is . . . something there. I'm so sure. I've even made questions I'm going to ask God when I see him, and he'd better give me some good answers," he said, smiling slyly.

"Do you think you're going to get to see him, then?" I asked.

He sighed. "Well, no. I don't really believe in God, but I don't think this life is for nothing. There is . . . something afterwards."

"Well, it's quite possible," I said.

"The only way you know is by dying."

"Aren't you afraid of dying?"

"No, but the way in which I die scares me. But once you know that you can decide yourself. . . . That's the important thing. . . . "

The next morning, John de Wit, the ward doctor, broached the subject with Dr. Edelman, the department head. Dr. Edelman was agitated. He said that he was too busy to make the preparations. Maybe someone else could do it. On the other hand, he knew David well and felt obliged to do it himself. But it was impossible this week, maybe next week. In the course of time, I had come to recognize this reaction. Dr. Edelman was struggling with the dilemma of relieving a patient's suffering by assisting in terminating his life. He was agitated because he knew that the request was justified and that he would not be able to refuse it. He needed time to adjust, emotionally. He asked John to talk to David; he would call in later.

Together with John, I went to David's room. John explained that they understood his situation, that they thought his request was justified, and that they were willing to help him, but that it wasn't something they could just decide overnight. Certain rules had to be followed. David listened in silence, nodding occasionally.

Later the same morning, Dr. Edelman also talked with David. I visited him in the afternoon. He was sitting next to the table, his feet up, heels resting on the edge of the bed. On the table was a packet of cigarettes, an ashtray containing a few cigarette butts and an open book. He was stirring his tea.

"I just stopped in to see how you were doing," I said.

"Oh, I'm all right," he answered. "I'm glad that everything has been arranged and I can relax now. It's a relief to know that it's all settled and that I have the certainty." He paused. "And I can always delay or cancel it if I change my mind. I hadn't expected it to be so complicated. I thought I could just ask for a cocktail and get it and take it when I wanted. I didn't realize there was so much that had to be arranged. I still have to wait a whole week. Every night when I go to bed I hope that I won't wake up again in the morning."

"What did you arrange with them? Tuesday?"

"Tuesday, Wednesday, Thursday. Edelman said sometime in the middle of the week. He wants to do it himself because he's known me for so long."

"Are you going to go home on the weekend?"

"No, no, I'm not going home." He fell silent. "There's no use going home now," he resumed after a few minutes. "And it's nice and quiet here, you know. It's good to think. I've been doing a lot of thinking. It's nice to sit and think by yourself. I've been asking myself a lot of questions, and giving myself all the answers. The nice thing about being by yourself is that you have all the answers." He looked at me slyly. "I give myself just the answers I want to hear." He laughed.

"You seem to be quite calm and philosophical about everything," I said. "Aren't you depressed?"

"Well, I can't really complain. I've had a good life. I've always had clothes on my back, enough to eat, enough money. I could have lived in worse circumstances. If I'd lived in Africa I would have been long dead by now. So altogether I'm satisfied."

"Don't you feel bitter at all?"

"Well, at first I thought I should be bitter, that I had to apportion blame. But I couldn't find anyone to blame or anything to be bitter about."

"What do you do the whole day? Do you just sit and think?"

"I read a lot."

"What do you read?"

"Stephen King. I really like Stephen King."

"What are you reading now?"

"*Thinner.*"

We went on to discuss Stephen King.

"You've almost finished the book," I said.

"Yes, last night I went to bed at nine o'clock, but after two minutes I had to get up again to finish the chapter. I couldn't wait until the next day to find out what happened. I've read all his books except one. Maybe I'll start that tomorrow, but I'm not sure whether I'll be able to finish it before Wednesday. It wouldn't do if I had to ask Edelman to postpone the euthanasia until I'd finished my book, would it?" He laughed.

"You know," he said, after another long silence, "I wonder what it's going to be like to die. I believe that there is something there after death. I don't believe that it just stops. I'm not religious or anything like that, though I was brought up as a Catholic, but I do think that we continue in some form after death. I don't know where, but by now it'll probably be very crowded."

I looked at him. His face was yellow, with blotches of Kaposi's sarcoma on his cheeks. His nose was black and lumpy. Outside, on the street or in the supermarket, he might have appeared monstrous, but in the context of the AIDS ward, he still seemed reasonably healthy. He wasn't emaciated, he wasn't bedridden, he wasn't blind, and he could still enjoy Stephen King. I had the sudden feeling that it was too soon for him to die, that it would be a loss.

"Don't you think you're still too well to die just yet?" I asked.

"I don't *feel* well."

"I mean, you can still read and walk around and enjoy things."

"I had a shower this morning and it almost finished me. I was exhausted by the time I finished. That's not how I want to go on."

That evening I sat at home and brooded. I decided not to go to the hospital the next day. But throughout Friday and Saturday I was haunted by the thought of David sitting there in his room, waiting. It depressed me. On Sunday I managed to repress all thought of David, but on Monday morning he was there again. I should have gone to the hospital, but I remained at home, unconsciously hoping that it would all be over when I did return, but at the same time feeling guilty about having deserted him.

On Tuesday I forced myself to go to the hospital. I couldn't just let him die without having said good-bye. I drove to the hospital and climbed the stairs to the AIDS ward. It was then that I ran into

Dr. Edelman in the corridor, and he told me that it was all arranged for later that morning.

When Dr. Edelman had disappeared around the corner I went into the ward. David's door was closed. I knocked.

"Come in," a voice called.

I poked my head around the door. "Am I disturbing you?" I asked.

"No," he said. "Come on in."

I sat down in the other chair. "How are you feeling?" I asked.

"All right," he said.

"How was your weekend?"

"It was okay."

"Did you go out of the hospital?"

"No. I didn't have the energy."

"Did you manage to finish your book?"

"Yes, I finished it," He smiled, "but I didn't start reading the other one in case I couldn't finish it in time."

"I just heard that it's all arranged for this morning," I said.

"Yes. My mother and brother are coming at eleven. Before that, Rob Edelman will come with the papers to sign, and then he'll bring the cocktail at eleven-thirty."

"You can always postpone it or cancel it if you change your mind," I said.

He paused to light a cigarette. "No, I can't postpone it," he said, smiling, as he held out his open cigarette pack. "I've only got enough cigarettes to last me till eleven-thirty. If I postpone, then I'll have to go downstairs again for a new pack."

"I admire your courage," I said.

"Don't speak too soon. I might not be so courageous when the time comes. No, but seriously, I've seen so many people suffer. I saw the guy in the room across there suffer. I don't want to suffer like that. What for? When you know you're going to die anyway."

"Yes, some people do hang on right to the bitter end," I said.

"Perhaps they don't have any belief." He fell silent, and we both stared out into the misty gloom of the winter morning.

"It's lousy weather for your last day," I said.

"No," he said, turning to look at me. "I think it's appropriate." He fell silent again.

"Last night," he said after a while, "I told myself it was just like going for an operation. Only I'd have to get washed and neatly dressed and take a small drink first." On his bed lay a pile of neatly folded clothes.

When his mother and brother arrived, I left. I returned just before Dr. Edelman was due to bring the fatal cocktail. This time David was sitting up in bed. He looked well-groomed. He had washed and neatly combed his hair and he wore a clean sweater. He looked tense. I walked up to the bed and stood next to him. What do you say to someone who is about to die?

"Well," I said nervously. "I've come to say good-bye."

He smiled.

"I just want to say again that I really admire your courage, and the way in which you've coped with everything. And not only me. Everyone here on the ward admires your courage." My throat contracted and the blood streamed to my head. I bit off my words, afraid that my voice would falter. I saw his eyes grow moist, and, for an instant, I had the feeling that we were both gripped in a single emotional force field. It was a few seconds before we regained our composure.

"We'll meet again, you know, afterward, even though you don't believe it." He smiled.

"I never said I didn't believe it," I replied. "I only said we couldn't know for sure. Anyway, you'll find out soon enough." I didn't know what else to say. I held out my hand. "Well, good-bye," I said. He shook my hand stiffly and his eyes gleamed moistly. I turned to go. His brother sat at the foot of the bed, crying. It was half past eleven.

In the dispensary, Dr. Edelman was busy grinding various pills in a small mortar. When he had finished, he swept the resulting powder into a glass with the edge of his hand. He looked up as I entered.

"I'm just preparing a cocktail for David," he said cheerfully. "I asked him what flavor he wanted and he chose orange." His mouth smiled, but his eyes were sad. It was a cheerfulness that I had come to recognize as masking deep despondency.

After he had dissolved the powder in some orange juice, he edged past me into the corridor. I followed and saw him disappear into David's room.

Now all we had to do was wait for death.

A few minutes later Dr. Edelman emerged and walked hurriedly down the corridor before disappearing through the swinging doors into the hall. He ignored me as he passed. Later he told me that David had drunk his cocktail in a single gulp, after having smoked his last cigarette.

"You're exactly on time," David had said when Dr. Edelman arrived. "I was down to my last cigarette."

It was while standing outside David's room that I suddenly became aware of my incongruous position. Wearing my white doctor's coat, I had always been inconspicuous in the hospital. Now, however, standing aimlessly in the corridor, I was out of place. What was I doing there anyway? What was my role? I wasn't a detached observer, not anymore, but I wasn't really relevant either. I had nothing to contribute medically. I wasn't a relative. I wasn't even a friend in any real sense of the word. Still, I was involved, more deeply and emotionally than I had thought possible.

I went into the doctors' office (all ward doctors share one office). It was empty. I paced back and forth. I went out into the corridor again. The ward secretary and one of the nurses were decorating a large Christmas tree with lights. David was already in a deep coma and his face had turned blue, one of the nurses told me. He was dying. Dr. Edelman had said it would take about an hour, but it was now an hour and a half since David had swallowed the cocktail, and his pulse was still strong.

I went back into the doctors' office and stood looking out the window at a city shrouded in cold fog. I sat down at the desk. On it lay David's medical record and a typed statement that read as follows:

> Since July 1991 I have been treating David Marner, born 17 September 1959 . . . [He's only thirty-three, I thought, four years younger than me] . . . he was diagnosed as having AIDS on the basis of sero-positivity for HIV-1, Kaposi's sarcoma, and recidivistic oral candida. . . . After three months of treatment with AZT the Kaposi's quickly became progressive. In July 1992 he received chemotherapy, but his condition deteriorated rapidly. He developed a very painful spinal infection. He

became progressively yellow as a result of an untreatable infection of the bile ducts. In the meantime the Kaposi's was progressive and disfigured his face and body . . .

So it continued up to the final paragraph:

Given his hopeless situation and at his own request, I, the undersigned, provided him with a euthanaticum [medication given by a doctor with the intention of euthanizing the patient] on the 15th of December at 11:30 a.m., as a result of which he died on the 15th of December 1992 at _____ o'clock.

Only the time needed to be filled in. The statement was signed Dr. R. Edelman.

I flipped open the cover of his dossier. A photograph fell out onto the desk. David was standing against a white background. His torso was bare, and the camera had been focused on the large blotches of Kaposi's sarcoma covering his abdomen. He had a peculiar smile on his face. "You are allowed to smile in medical photos, if you want," I imagined the hospital photographer saying. It was the kind of smile you would give in response to a remark such as that.

Another hour passed before David's pulse stopped and I could go home, broken.

For me, David's death was, symbolically, the last in almost two years of anthropological research on the social context in which euthanasia decisions are made. During my research, I saw more than fifty people die, their deaths often preceded by the extended agony of debilitating disease, horrible symptoms, and physical decay, sometimes also by loneliness or emotional drama. David's death was not literally the last death that I experienced in the course of my research. After his death, however, I realized that I had had enough. I was tired, both physically and mentally, of the balancing act between involvement and detachment that is called anthropological fieldwork.

EMOTION AND THE ANTHROPOLOGY OF DEATH

When the social sciences study death, they usually do so from a distance, dividing its various aspects so that they fit into existing disciplinary categories. Anthropologists almost never address dying (how people die), or their own emotional involvement in the death-related topics they describe. Palgi and Abramovitch note that "when reading through the literature in one large sweep, one is left with the impression of coolness and remoteness. The focus is on the bereaved and on the corpse but never on the dying" (Palgi and Abramovitch 1984:385). This observation was made over fifteen years ago but, with a few notable exceptions (Hockey 1990), is still true today.

In the social sciences, writing about the emotional involvement of the researcher is generally considered taboo, and in anthropology, any discussion of personal involvement is often relegated to what is contemptuously described as confession ethnography. However, as Mary-Louise Pratt (1986) has pointed out, such involvement in fact forms an integral part of the way in which anthropologists understand and interpret other cultures. Personal narratives have always been part of ethnography because they are necessary to bridge the contradiction between direct personal encounters in the field and the norms of an impersonal scientific discourse, but they are usually relegated to the margins of formal ethnographic description, to notes, introductions, and appendixes. Ethnographers, Pratt continues,

> leave out or hopelessly impoverish some of the most important knowledge they have achieved, including self-knowledge. For the lay person, such as myself, the main evidence of a problem is the simple fact that ethnographic writing tends to be surprisingly boring. How, one asks constantly, could such interesting people doing such interesting things produce such dull books? What did they have to do to themselves? (Pratt 1986:33)

This absence is most striking in the anthropology of death. Renato Rosaldo has remarked that "in a manner peculiarly at odds with the intense emotions it arouses, the topic of death has proven a particularly fertile area in the production of distanced normalizing accounts" (Rosaldo 1989:55). According to Rosaldo, the experience of intense emotion and concomitant personal development can enhance anthropological understanding. In "Grief and the Headhunter's Rage," he shows how the sudden death of his wife, who fell down a precipice to her death during fieldwork in the Philippines, made it possible for him to understand why anger resulting from the loss of a loved one drove Ilongots to take heads: "Immediately on finding her body I became enraged. How could she abandon me? How could she have been so stupid as to fall? I tried to cry. I sobbed, but rage blocked the tears" (Rosaldo 1989:9).

Opening this book with a description of David's death is not intended to give the impression that, in my research on euthanasia, I was emotionally involved with all patients. In fact, I was not. As in the social interaction of ordinary life, my involvement with those with whom I worked varied. Sometimes we hit it off immediately, but more often we did not. With most patients the relationship was cordial and open, with some it was more intimate, while with others it was distant. What is perhaps most striking about my relationships with those I studied is that they were not *more* distant: I only experienced one frank refusal during two years of research. This surprised me, especially when I took the time to speculate on how I would react if I were terminally ill and some anthropologist showed up wanting to study how I was to die.

I have opened this presentation with David because I think that emotion and the personal involvement of the researcher are undervalued in social scientific studies of death. I did not want to reduce the emotionally charged deaths of people such as David to dull and neutral descriptions of social processes. I also wanted to show that the research process is a praxis in which the researcher is an integral part, and in which personal, emotional, and irrational factors play a role. But perhaps, if I am completely honest with myself, I also opened with a patient with whom I was emotionally involved to soothe my own conscience about being less emotionally touched by the suffering and deaths of others. I had sympathized with all patients, even pitied some, but I had not always felt real empathy, and this disturbed me. Differences of class, generation, and personality all played a role, but the chasm that separated me most fundamentally from the patients and their relatives—both those with whom I was personally involved and those with whom I was not—was the fact that they were dying, or about to lose a loved one—I was not.

PARTICIPANT OBSERVATION

How does one go about studying a topic such as this? During 1990 to 1991 a large national survey was carried out to investigate the nature and incidence of euthanasia in the Netherlands, with a view to developing new legislation (Van der Maas, Van Delden, and Pijnenborg, 1991). Although doctors were generally considered to have been open in their responses to the questionnaires, partly due to guarantees from the Ministry of Justice that no prosecutions would follow from information revealed during the survey, it was still generally acknowledged that relatively little was known about how euthanasia decisions were reached, in practice, and what kind of role social contextual factors played in these decisions. Participant observation seemed to me the only way to get this information.

Participant observation implies that the researcher joins the group to be studied—traditionally another culture—and participates in its activities. The researcher is always around to observe first-hand what group members are doing, and having done this for an extended period of time, often several years, he or she is able to form a picture of the culture and to develop an understanding of what the members of that culture are doing and why. The participant observer is, simultaneously, both an insider, viewing things through the eyes of the natives, and an outsider, noticing and critically appraising actions and explanations that are taken for granted by the natives, placing them in a wider context, and thus generating understanding.

This is, of course, the stereotypical view of participant observation, which has been criticized to such an extent that it has become almost cliché. The extent to which outside anthropologists can "really" participate in the lives of people in another culture has been questioned. Anthropologists often do not speak the vernacular fluently; they come from a different ethnic, cultural, or class background; and they may lack the cultural competence necessary to properly interpret what is happening around them.

These considerations notwithstanding, the basic fact of fieldwork seems to be simply that the ethnographer is *there*, tagging along, looking, listening, poking his or her nose in wherever possible, and asking questions. For me, one of the basic assumptions was that relevant and interesting information about euthanasia was more likely to surface in informal contexts than in formal interview settings. To get that information, I needed to be present. This was easier said than done, however, and getting access to a suitable medical institution was a major problem.

When I was planning this study, a doctor said to me, referring to previous research I had done on witchcraft in Cameroon, "If you think it was difficult getting admitted to secret societies in West Africa, wait until you try to gain access to the medical institutions here in the Netherlands; that's *really* difficult." He was right. This reluctance was, of course, largely due to the delicate nature of the topic. Euthanasia was, and still is, illegal in the Netherlands as well as a rewarding topic for sensationalism. Doctors were worried, quite rightly, about exposing their patients and themselves to the media and the risk of legal proceedings.

Such justifiable reservations, however, were not the only impediment. In some of the institutions that I approached, my proposal was eagerly utilized as a means of fighting out all manner of petty internal squabbles. If I approached the director of a hospital who was enthusiastic about the proposed research, but happened to have a conflict with the medical staff about something completely different, then the latter would oppose the research unconditionally, and if the specialists supported the research but happened to have a conflict with the nursing staff, then the nurses would make use of their veto to emphasize their independence vis-à-vis the doctors. All this emerged later through informal enquiries.

It finally became clear that formal approaches would not work and that access to a hospital would only be possible through a network of personal contacts. It was also clear that the specialists were the most important point of access. If the specialists wanted the research and everyone else was opposed, I would still have a chance, albeit small, but if everyone was enthusiastic about the research and the specialists were opposed then I would have no chance at all.

At this point, a member of the project's steering committee, and later minister of health, introduced me to Dr. Edelman, an internist at the Randstad Hospital,[2] a 400-bed teaching hospital situated in Randstad, the large conurbation spread along the west coast of Holland, stretching from Amsterdam in the north to Rotterdam in the south. Dr. Edelman was too busy to participate in the research, he said, but the proposal looked interesting, and because he had great respect for the committee member in question, he decided to introduce me to the hospital psychologist, Marthe Diepen.

Ms. Diepen was enthusiastic about the project and convened a meeting with two specialists with whom she had close contact: Dr. Nieuwenhuis, a gastroenterologist, and Dr. Glas, a pulmonologist. We discussed the project one afternoon and they were interested. They said that I could accompany them provisionally during consultations and rounds, until the hospital's ethics committee had approved my proposal and the director had granted formal permission. After eight months, I had finally made it.

PERFORMATIVE ETHNOGRAPHY

One of the most important objections to participant observation is that the data produced may be biased. To prevent this, it is often argued that researchers should try to exclude their own views and preconceptions so as not to "contaminate" their model of what the people they are studying are doing (see, e.g., Saville-Troike 1982: 121; Kleinman 1980:25-26). Another important objection focuses on the problem of "informant accuracy"—that different informants may say different things about the same topic (Bernard et al. 1984; Freeman, Romney, and Freeman, 1987; Heider 1988). These problems are, however, only apparent. They are based on untenable assumptions about the nature of social processes, social knowledge, everyday communication, our attempts to study these factors, and our resulting scientific knowledge.

Social researchers always influence the reality they study: recording conversations, or simply the presence of a researcher or a tape recorder, influences what people say, how they say it, and how they act (Tedlock 1983; Pool 1994). During the first weeks of my research on euthanasia, I thought, perhaps somewhat naively, that I would be relatively inconspicuous in my white coat among the doctors and medical students. I sat next to the doctors during consultations, and I accompanied them on their rounds. I was there when the doctor informed a patient of his or her diagnosis and prognosis, and I was present when treatment options were discussed with colleagues. They knew, of course, that I was there and what I was doing, but I assumed that they would soon get used to my presence and not, as far as their decision making was concerned, take any notice of me. This is what I thought, that is, until I began to encounter my name in the case notes.

One day I read, "The patient has expressed the desire for euthanasia. Robert Pool will discuss this with him this afternoon. We await his findings." The doctors started to ask me for my opinion on certain euthanasia requests, and, on the odd occasion, I was asked to write reports in patients' case notes. I had become an expert. I was relatively neutral, I was familiar with all those involved, I knew the various points of view, and I had an overview of the whole social situation. I had plenty of time to discuss a particular euthanasia process at leisure with all those involved and was in a good position to identify misunderstandings, to place apparently contradictory statements, actions, and interpretations in their wider context. I could not refuse to contribute, and, as a result, I could not avoid influencing what I was studying. This is not a methodological flaw that must be hidden, but an integral aspect of this kind of social research that we must accept and make explicit in the presentation of results.

Variations in accounts and explanations of the same situation by different respondents (and even by the same respondent at different times) and a degree of indeterminacy, particularly in relation to situations characterized by uncertainty and ambiguity, are also an integral part of qualitative social research. Some forms of knowledge, such as technical knowledge, are highly systematized, and practical activities based on that knowledge are relatively rational and predictable. In other domains, less systematic social knowledge plays a greater role and actions are determined to a far greater extent by contingent factors such as situation, mood, personality, and implicit communication. In such cases, it may be difficult for those involved to explain why they acted as they did, or to make the rules governing their actions fully explicit. It is on the latter type of factors that this book focuses.

The type of qualitative social research on which this book is based is not a process in which objective data are gathered by applying the proper methods, and interviews are not seen simply as a means of information transfer. The traditional distinction between data and interpretation is untenable because the decision as to what will count as data is already the result of interpretation. In this context, Fabian speaks of *performative* as opposed to *informative* ethnography. Sometimes the information that the researcher wants is not there, in people's heads, ready to be called up and expressed in discursive statements that can then be collected and taken home as "data": it has to be made present through enactment, performance:

> In fact, once one sees matters in this light, the answers we get to our ethnographic questions can be interpreted as so many cultural performances. Cultural knowledge is always mediated by "acting." Performances . . . although they can be asked for, are not really responses to questions. The ethnographer's role, then, is no longer that of questioner; he or she is but a provider of occasions, a catalyst in the weakest sense, and a producer in the strongest. (Fabian 1990:6-7)

In this sense, the discussions I had with doctors and patients about euthanasia can be seen as "performances," as the making present of cultural knowledge. My presence acted as a catalyst, forcing the participants to reflect on and make explicit what they were doing and why (see Chapter 6).

The concept of performance, however, is also relevant in another sense. This book is based largely on ten detailed case studies, each featuring a patient, his or her relatives, doctors, nurses, and an anthropologist. It is useful to conceptualize these case studies as performances as well. Each performance, or complex of actions, utterances, and decisions, centers around a euthanasia request (or related end-of-life decision) and continues until the patient dies and the group of individuals brought together by the request disintegrates. The information and the interpretations that are relevant are generated through this praxis; they are actualized in practical situations, in performances (Fabian 1990; Pool 1994). This book can be seen as a presentation of a number of such performances, accompanied by interpretations and discussion.

Chapter 2

Euthanasia According to the Rules

THE ENDOSCOPY ROOM

During my first weeks at the hospital, I spent most of my time in the endoscopy room. The endoscope is an instrument that enables the gastroenterologist to examine the stomach and intestines of his or her patients. It consists of a long flexible hose, the tip of which is slipped through the sphincter and guided up through the rectum and into the colon or, alternatively, down the esophagus and into the stomach. The tip holds a light; a lens, so the gastroenterologist can see possible abnormalities through a viewer or on a video screen; a water jet, to wash away traces of feces; and a small claw, to remove pieces of suspect tissue for further analysis.

On most mornings, Dr. Nieuwenhuis, the gastroenterologist, received patients in the endoscopy room. After a briefing, the patient was wheeled over to the endoscope, and Dr. Nieuwenhuis, protected by a plastic apron, made his journey through the colon or esophagus. When he was finished, he discussed his findings with the patient and, after the patient left, wrote a report before the next patient arrived.

I followed Dr. Nieuwenhuis's journeys through the gastrointestinal tracts of his patients on the video screen, I listened to his briefings and debriefings, and I sat quietly in the corner while he wrote his reports.

"There's a woman on the internal ward who's requested euthanasia," Dr. Nieuwenhuis said one morning, pausing from his report writing. "Her name is Mrs. Kees. Mark Hansen, the junior doctor attending her, has asked me for a second opinion. I think you should have a talk with him. Do you want me to introduce you?"

I nodded and he picked up the phone. He explained my research briefly and asked Dr. Hansen whether I could come to see him. He then passed the phone to me, and I made an appointment for later that day.

THE ATTENDING PHYSICIAN

Dr. Hansen was waiting for me when I walked onto the internal ward at the appointed time. We went into his office.

"Ah, yes, Mrs. Kees," he said, even before we were seated. As I was to find out on countless occasions, more important matters were pressing and he had no time for informal chatter. "She was referred to me with abdominal symptoms. Later, one of her friends told me that she had been vomiting for a year and a half and had lost a lot of weight. When she was admitted, we looked in her stomach but it wasn't yet possible to confirm that there was a malignity. But, given the results of the radiological examination, the CT [computerized tomography] scan and the X rays, we suspected a malignity. A physical examination revealed a tumor in the lower abdomen. We weren't sure whether it was a metastasis of the stomach tumor. She also had ascite . . . ascites is fluid in the abdominal cavity, you know. Then we did an ascitic fluid tap and found cancer cells. And, well, that meant that she had a peritoneal carcinomatosis, which means that the cancer had spread throughout the abdomen.

"So, I gave her the diagnosis and I told her that we still didn't know the exact significance of the tumor in her stomach. I told her that the surgeon wanted to try and make a bypass. While we were discussing the possibilities she introduced her euthanasia request. And how did that come about? Her husband had died of lung cancer five years previously. He had a euthanasia declaration, but they had never told anybody about it. Their GP [general practitioner] was also unaware of it, and when they told him at that late stage, he would have nothing of it. She was scared that if she turned out to have cancer and her condition deteriorated, the same thing might happen to her. She wanted to make her ideas regarding euthanasia clear to as many people as possible in an early stage."

I asked Mark whether she had broached the topic directly or indirectly, explicitly or implicitly.

"No, she didn't ask me directly in the first instance," he said. "Her son and daughter came to see me. I told them, 'Don't expect me to broach the topic with her. That's something the patient has to do herself.' So then the next day during rounds, she said that she had a euthanasia declaration and asked whether we would honor her request if she asked for euthanasia."

"Did she actually use the word euthanasia?" I asked.

"Yes, yes, yes. And she's very persistent, you know. She's had her operation in the meantime. They couldn't do anything with the tumor in the stomach, but the surgeon made a bypass round the tumor in the lower abdomen—that's the one at the beginning of the small intestine—they made a detour to the stomach. Apart from that, they did nothing. She was full of tumor, all metastases. Really, it was . . . it was horrible . . . . "

"Did she discuss her euthanasia request with you again later?"

"Yes. She said that she had expected as much. Her mother had died of stomach cancer. The symptoms had been exactly the same. She had taken care of her mother, so she knew that she had the same thing."

"What did she say about euthanasia?"

"Last Wednesday she wanted euthanasia that very day. I'm not sure exactly what she expected. She said, 'I'd rather do it today.' She was also a bit panicky because she goes from one pain peak to another, you know. By accident, she hadn't received enough codeine the evening before, so she was in pain. She broke right through. So the next day she broached the topic. I said, 'Why don't we just wait a week?' She still had to discuss her request with other doctors because you can't just do it like that. You can't."

"So what happens next, in cases like that, generally speaking? Who is consulted and who isn't? How do you go about it here in this hospital?"

"The usual thing here is that you ask a couple of colleagues from various disciplines, colleagues who are not directly involved in the treatment of the patient, to talk to her. I've asked the psychologist, the anesthetist, and the gastroenterologist. And then, if you decide to carry it out, you have to report it to the director. So last Friday I went to see him. Well, he took note, and that's all. And as to what happens next, well, there are different opinions. Some say that you have to report your intention to the public prosecutor beforehand; others say that if you do that then you're reporting a crime that you haven't yet committed, and what's the public prosecutor supposed to do with that knowledge? So it seems better to do it first and then report that the death wasn't natural."

"If it's carried out, who will do it. You?"

"No, the anesthetist does that here."

"So she has to report it to the public prosecutor?"

"No, the attending physician has to do that. First, I thought that the director would report it because, in the final instance, it's the hospital's responsibility. But that isn't the case; it's the attending physician who is responsible."

"What do you think will happen next? Do you think it will take place on Wednesday or, . . . ? What do you think?"

"This woman is very persistent; she wants euthanasia at all costs . . . . I only mentioned Wednesday, but she's keeping me to it. She's looking forward to it. I think it's a good thing that different people talk to her so that you get a good picture and know for sure that it's not an empty request stemming from depression or not being able to cope with the diagnosis."

"I read somewhere in case notes, 'Does she want to or doesn't she?' with lots of question marks."

"Yes, yes. . . . When she talks to me her request is consistent, but when she talks to the nurses she sometimes says things like, 'Well, I'm not in pain right now, and I can still see the children, so . . . I can still hold out for a while. I would like to live a bit longer.' But then when I come along, or the internist, then she really wants it to go ahead on Wednesday. But we keep emphasizing, 'Even if it's one minute before, if you change your mind, don't do it. You just have to say the word and we'll stop everything.' "

"Have you discussed it with her GP?"

"That's a good question: no. She recently changed to another GP. He hardly knows her, but, yes, we should call him."

"You said the anesthetist carries it out. Does that mean that she's often involved in cases like this?"

"Yes, I think that the anesthetist—well, at least here in this hospital—is generally the one who actually carries it out."

"Does she know the patients, or does she just carry it out under instructions from the attending physician?"

"No, she knows a lot about the patient. It's not just. . . . She really helps in the decision making, as much as is necessary. She's also a doctor who has to act professionally. . . ."

"Is Mrs. Kees religious?"

"No."

"Do you think she'd be willing to talk to me about her euthanasia request, or do you think it's a bit too delicate?"

"Well, we can ask her. You'll just have to ask her. It is something that keeps her occupied at the moment: it's not long now, you know."

"In cases like this I would like to talk to the patient and her family as much as possible, but I don't want to start with people who can't cope, emotionally."

"She's very open . . . you know. I think you could easily talk to her. But I think I'll introduce you first. I'll go and ask her what she thinks about it."

"Yes, if you would."

"Okay, I'll try."

"Shall I phone you later then, or stop in?"

"No, I'll go and see her right now. If you wait a moment, I'll be right back." He stood up and disappeared through the door.

A feeling of panic gradually rose in my abdomen. I had been in the hospital two weeks and, up until now, had only seen patients from a relative distance, my limited interaction with them always mediated by others. Wearing my white coat, I had always blended in among the doctors and medical students during rounds, and in the endoscopy room, the patients had been much too preoccupied to notice me in my corner. Now, suddenly, without preparation, I was considering talking to a terminally ill woman about her reasons for not wanting to live any longer. What do I ask someone in that position? How do I ask the questions? How do I justify occupying someone's last moments, not to help that person (I didn't even have that legitimacy), but to do my research, write my book, and, ultimately, develop my career? I didn't know.

MRS. KEES

Mark returned, interrupting my speculation. It was okay, he said. Her son, Gerard, was present, and they had both agreed to see me.

We walked down the corridor to her room. Mark introduced me, and then silence descended as they all looked at me expectantly.

"Mark said that you wanted to talk to me," I said nervously.

"No, no, no," Mark said, agitated. "Mrs. Kees has given you *permission* to talk to her."

"Yes, of course," I said. "That's what I meant, that you were willing to talk to me."

"Oh no, here it comes again," Mrs. Kees said suddenly, leaning forward with difficulty, supported by her son, and vomiting into a stainless steel kidney dish. Strings of mucus joined her mouth to the dish.

"Sorry," she said, looking at me between convulsions of retching, "I don't think I'll be able to manage our talk today. Maybe we can try again tomorrow." She fell back onto her pillow, pale and exhausted, and lay there motionless, with her eyes closed.

I said that it didn't matter and that I would return some other time. I turned to leave, thankfully, and Gerard followed. He said that he wanted to talk to me, and we walked to the lounge together in silence.

THE SON

"My mother's choice has to be seen against the background of the death of my father," Gerard said, when we had settled down at a table with a cup of coffee. "He died of cancer about five and a half years ago. The whole disease process lasted for five years. He had lung cancer and they removed a lung. Then he developed metastases in a kidney. They removed that as well, but then they discovered cancer in the other kidney. He was very sober about it all; he decided to stop all treatment and go home. It was all a terrible burden on my mother. My father had signed a euthanasia declaration, but they hadn't told anybody about it. So the GP wasn't aware of it, and when they told him, he wasn't willing to do it. When my mother became ill, she was terribly afraid that if it was cancer and it became unbearable, the doctors would also refuse to help her. That's why she wanted to inform as many people as possible in an early stage."

I asked him about his family background.

"My parents weren't religious, and my sister and I didn't receive a religious education, so euthanasia fits rather well in our philosophy of life. We've always had the idea that clinging onto life when you're that far gone is quite useless. . . . " He fell silent. "Although," he resumed after a while, "when she decided to fix a date, even though she wasn't really suffering or in a hopeless—no, hopeless isn't the right word because it *was* hopeless—when she was in a . . . relatively . . . bearable condition, I thought it was rather absurd. It's her right, of course, to want it—there's no doubt about that—but perhaps it would be more suitable to increase the morphine gradually, when the moment arrives. . . .

"We weren't religious, and we sometimes discussed these things. I also have a declaration. . . . I've had it for the last twenty years. It's all quite compatible with the family philosophy. I know that my mother thinks very deeply about such matters. She never attended secondary school, but she did read a lot. I always used to think that she should have done something more than just staying home as a housewife. So she has thought about it carefully. After the operation, she really wanted to be fully conscious; that's her character.

"I was always her favorite, so I have the feeling that I understand her. She didn't want to find herself in a situation over which she didn't have control. That's why they reduced the morphine. But then the pain became unbearable. I remember that, on that Monday, she asked the doctor to do it right there and then, but he said, 'Well, that's a bit hasty. Why don't we agree on next Wednesday, then we have the time to discuss and say our good-byes.' I don't think that that really makes much difference; they might as well have done it last week. . . .

"Actually, my mother and I parted emotionally a long time ago, so there's no need for that now. . . . We knew someone who was going to have euthanasia, and, all of a sudden, her children all returned home and they talked for hours and hours, and they said, 'Now we've got a mother again.' I don't need that. I've already said what I want to say, and so has my sister, so there's no need for repeating it now."

THE PSYCHOLOGIST

After my discussion with Gerard, I called in to see the psychologist, Marthe Diepen. I told her that I had been to see Mrs. Kees but had been unable to talk to her. I asked her what she knew of Mrs. Kees's euthanasia request.

"When they decided to operate, she was afraid that if she went into a coma, then they might keep her alive as a plant. Mark Hansen asked me to talk to her on the day before the operation. She told me that she wasn't sure what she had, but that she suspected cancer. Her mother and her husband had both died of cancer, so she had experience with the disease. She had already discussed her desire for euthanasia with her children, and she had a euthanasia declaration so that she couldn't be kept alive artificially against her will. Her children both have euthanasia declarations.

"At her own request, I made a photocopy of her euthanasia declaration and put it in her case notes. Then I explained the options to her. She could gradually fall into a deep sleep and then into a coma by increasing the amount of pain medication, after which any arrangements which had been made would be implemented. Or she could continue with less morphine and more pain, remaining relatively clear minded, and then perhaps have her euthanasia request granted when the pain became really unbearable. She chose the second option.

"Immediately after the operation they gave her morphine, which made her sleepy. This was stopped because she didn't want to be sleepy. After the operation she was calmer and less nauseous.

"Mark phoned me in the middle of last week to inform me that an appointment for euthanasia had been arranged for the coming Wednesday. He asked me if I could go and talk to Mrs. Kees as part of the procedure. I told him it wasn't necessary because he already had a second opinion. He asked me whether he should report it beforehand. I didn't know because the guidelines had just changed, and I told him to ask the director. He was going to report what he was planning to do to the director anyway. I don't know how that turned out.

"Then I went to see Mrs. Kees. She was lucid and confirmed the arrangements. They had agreed on Wednesday because she wanted to speak to her children. I gave the flowers some water; they'd wilted. She said, 'I'm using you to water the flowers for me.' I said, 'It's good to be able to do something for you.' I sat down next to her bed. I said, 'What a job, being sick.' She said, 'You're right.' I didn't write anything in the case notes; there was nothing new to report. I didn't see the children."

"You mentioned a second opinion," I said. "I gathered that the anesthetist was going to talk to her because she was the one who was actually going to carry it out."

"Yes," said Marthe, and she hesitated. "That's always a bit unclear, you know. Actually, the attending specialist should do that because he bears ultimate responsibility. But, in practice, the anesthetist often inserts the intravenous line because she has experience in doing that. She also often decides on the appropriate dosage. In theory, the attending specialist should open the tap, though."

"Isn't Mark the attending specialist?" I asked.

"No, he is the attending *physician*. Van Ham is probably the attending *specialist*, and he is unapproachable when it comes to that topic. That may be the reason why Mark is doing it in the first place. I noticed that Mark was playing a central role in this, and I'm not sure whether he's doing it in consultation with Van Ham. In the guidelines [the hospital ethics committee's recommendations regarding euthanasia], it states that the responsibility for euthanasia can't be delegated, but as far as the law is concerned, Mark *is allowed* to do it." Marthe fell silent and stared in front of her.

"In any case," she resumed after a while, "she was very positive about the ward and how she had been cared for. She appreciated having her own room and that everyone was pleasant and patient. That makes a big difference. And the arrangements gave her peace. She fully trusted everyone. The nursing staff didn't avoid her, which sometimes happens when dying patients are put in separate rooms. But she also isn't any trouble. She prefers to do everything herself. She values her independence and her right to decide for herself highly. When I visited her, she was too weak to put the euthanasia declaration back into her bag. I did it for her. She didn't get angry or anything like that, but I could see that she would have preferred to do it herself."

THE SECOND OPINION

That evening, when I picked up my coat in the endoscopy room, I saw that Dr. Nieuwenhuis was still in his office. I went in to tell him what I had been doing. I had spent the whole day discussing Mrs. Kees's euthanasia request.

"Yes, Mrs. Kees," he said. "That's someone who really wants euthanasia, and who's thought about it for a long time. I had a pithy discussion with her on Friday. She didn't like it. But I didn't know her, and I seriously wanted to find out whether she was doing it for the children or because she was depressive, or lonely, or something like that. If you give a patient nice music, the relatives come and visit more frequently, and the nurses are more friendly, then maybe the desire for euthanasia will disappear. It sounds a bit coarse, but sometimes you have the impression that it's really like that, and if you don't know the patient, then you have to eliminate that possibility and make sure that the request is genuine. And in her case, I think it is. She's very sick, and she has the right to request it. In this case, it's the junior doctor who is going to carry it out because he knows her well. I think that Van Ham, the specialist, wants to keep out of sight because he is opposed to euthanasia but doesn't want to stand in the way either."

DR. VAN HAM

My one, and only, discussion with Dr. Van Ham, Mrs. Kees's attending specialist, went as follows:

"I'm doing some research on decision making relating to euthanasia and I —"

"I'm opposed to euthanasia, so there is no euthanasia in my department; I don't allow it. So you're wasting your time."

"But why . . . ?"

"Why? Because the Pope has forbidden it, that's why. Good afternoon." He had placed his hand on my back and was guiding me lightly, but unmistakably, toward the door of his office.

"Can I come and talk to you about your reasons for opposing euthanasia?" I asked, in a last desperate attempt to maintain some kind of contact. He stopped suddenly and glared at me fiercely.

"Do you know how many journalists phone me every week asking for interviews? I've published a lot of articles, you know, and I've got a PhD. And those are not just ordinary journalists," he continued, before I had a chance to open my mouth. "They're *foreign* journalists, and they're willing to pay a lot of money for an interview with me. But I refuse to be interviewed because I'm too busy. Good afternoon." He held the door open.

THE HEAD NURSE

The next morning, Tuesday, I spoke to Inge, the head nurse of the general internal ward.

"How did the present situation relating to Mrs. Kees's euthanasia request develop?" I asked. "I gathered that on Wednesday—"

"Yes, she arranged that last week," Inge replied. "After the operation she was tired and sleepy. She told me then that whatever happened, she didn't want to be like that. On the weekend she was in a lot of pain, and we increased the codeine, but I don't think it's enough now. She's becoming restless. Yesterday she said, 'It's already Monday, not long to Wednesday now.' I thought, 'Oh no,' and I told her that we had medicines that would enable her to go gradually. But she immediately said that wasn't what she wanted; she wanted to remain conscious and as lucid as possible."

"Is she starting to hesitate now that the moment is nearing?" I asked.

"Yes . . . I don't know. I asked her directly whether she had second thoughts. She said, 'On the one hand I do, because I want to live, though only if I can be healthy. But whether it happens today or tomorrow, I'm going to die anyway, so then it's better to do it my way.' I always have the feeling . . . I mean. . . . She's realistic, but at the same time, it's so definitive, as though she thinks, 'I'd better go ahead, the children are coming, etc.' I told her that she can still always say 'No.' But that's something that Mrs. Kees doesn't want to do."

"I read in her file that she wants euthanasia but that she has told some of the nurses that she can always call it off at the last moment if she changes her mind. Underneath someone had written, 'Does she want to or doesn't she?'"

"Yes, that was Mieke Van der Ven, the anesthetist. I read it and then I confronted Mrs. Kees with it. She told me that she wanted to stick to the Wednesday. That was yesterday. I'm not sure whether it's such a good idea to make an appointment for a specific day like that, but it's already been done."

"Isn't it possible that she's started to hesitate but is continuing nonetheless because she thinks she's becoming a burden?" I asked.

"No, no. She says, 'I'm very egotistical: if I want something then I get it.' I keep telling her that she can change her mind at any time, even if her children are here, but she doesn't want to."

"What do you think about it?"

"I think she's right. She doesn't have much chance, no chance in fact, and even if she doesn't go ahead with it, she won't live for more than a couple of weeks at most. She's deteriorating fast, and in those last weeks, she will become progressively more drowsy as we increase the pain medication, which we'll have to do. What good will that do her? I wouldn't like to do it myself, but that's another story."

"So she wouldn't experience much pain without euthanasia?"

"No, because we'd increase the pain medication, though she doesn't want us to do that now. It's very brave of her."

"Why does she want to do it like this?"

"She doesn't want to deteriorate, in particular, mentally. And she doesn't want to just hang on to a numbed existence between the shots of morphine."

"Does the experience with her husband . . . ?"

"Yes, of course."

"Did she tell you that?"

"Not explicitly, but that's what I've read between the lines. She talks to her children a lot about that. They support her decision."

"How long has she been here on the ward?"

"Six weeks. We brought her back purposely after the operation. In cases like that, patients usually stay on the surgical ward. I discussed it with the team because I didn't think that would be a good idea. We know her well. So we brought her back after the operation. Everyone agreed."

"Wouldn't she prefer to die at home?"

"We discussed that yesterday. She said, 'No, that would put too much of a burden on the children. I can't do that to them. Home care is only eight hours a day. That means that there are still sixteen hours that the children have to take care of me. That's too much.' She's quite sure of what she wants and doesn't want. The only thing that she's hesitant about, perhaps, is the exact moment."

"When did she raise the issue of euthanasia for the first time?"

"Before her operation. She was angry because she thought that they would carry out the euthanasia the next day, on Saturday, as soon as they knew it was malignant. I was here on Sunday and discussed it with her. She didn't request it explicitly. She would have preferred to have died during the operation, then she wouldn't have known."

"Is there much euthanasia on this ward?"

"No, this is the first case in eleven years. Usually they just fade away under the pain medication."

"So if she had never mentioned euthanasia . . . ?"

"Then we would have given her more morphine sooner, and she would have just faded away by herself."

"Does everyone on the ward agree with what's happening?"

"Yes, but that's not always the case. The nurses are usually more in favor of withdrawing active treatment than the doctors. It also depends on the specialization involved. In this department [general internal medicine], there are a lot of old people with the prospect of spending their final days in a nursing home. In such cases, you're much more likely to listen to the wishes of the relatives. If the patient develops pneumonia, and they say, 'He would never have wanted this,' then we tend not to treat it. If they want us to treat it, then we treat it."

THE DAUGHTER

After my discussion with the head nurse, I went to the lounge where I had an appointment with Elizabeth, Mrs. Kees's daughter. Elizabeth was a woman in her thirties. She was accompanied by her husband, Karel, and brother, Gerard, to whom I had spoken the previous day. After shaking hands, I sat down.

While I was taking my cassette recorder out of my bag, Elizabeth said, "My mother doesn't want to talk about euthanasia anymore. This morning she said that the date was fixed and everything was arranged so there was no need to talk about it anymore. As far as she's concerned, she doesn't even need to talk to the doctors anymore. She knows what's in store for her and that's enough. She's had a euthanasia declaration for a long time; she signed it together with my father when he was sick."

"What played a role in that decision?" I asked. "Was it fear of pain and physical deterioration?"

"Asphyxiation," Elizabeth said.

"And just being sick for too long," Karel added.

"And what about now?" I asked. "Because I understand your mother is not in any real pain at the moment."

"It's the vomiting, the retching, and the fear that the pain is still to come. She doesn't want to just lie there and wait for it," Elizabeth said.

"She had that operation to stop the retching," Karel said, "but now it's started again, and that has made the decision easier for her."

"And the surgeon said that the bypass in her stomach won't last for long, and when that goes, she'll be in a lot of pain," Elizabeth said.

"What do *you* think of her decision?" I asked.

"Brave, very brave," Elizabeth said.

"Justified," Karel added. "We're also members of the Association [Association for Voluntary Euthanasia]. My own mother recently suffered a stroke. . . . It makes you think about it, but you delay. You think, 'I'm still young; I have time.' Things like this just speed up what you were already planning to do for a long time."

"But if it's possible to still the pain, why not die naturally?" I asked.

"If you've only got a few weeks left, why sit around and wait for more misery?" Karel asked.

"What value does life still have?" Elizabeth asked. "For her, it doesn't have any value anymore. But what I do find strange is the date. Usually you don't know the exact moment that someone is going to die—"

"You can anticipate it," Karel interrupted.

"Yes, but you never know exactly. *We know:* Wednesday, half past one. When we come to the hospital, we know that we're coming for *that.* It seems so strange."

"I mentioned that yesterday," Gerard said, looking across at me. "That it seems absurd . . . that you wonder: has she really reached the limit of what she can bear . . . ?"

"That's for her to decide," Elizabeth interjected fiercely.

"We can't set that limit for her," Karel added.

"She has a strong character," Elizabeth said. "We notice it all the time. She's terribly dominant, wants to arrange everything herself. This has also been arranged just as she wants it." Karel and Gerard nodded in agreement.

EUTHANASIA

On Wednesday, at half past twelve, I met Karel in the elevator. It was one hour before Mrs. Kees's euthanasia. I wasn't sure how to act. Should I smile, or would that be out of place? Karel was leaning against the wall of the elevator. He smiled easily and said hello. When the doors opened, I wished him good luck and walked into the hall. Gerard and Elizabeth sat on one of the sofas, smoking. They smiled and waved as I walked past.

In the doctor's office, Mark Hansen was nervously rummaging through the untidy piles of papers and files. He did not look up when I entered and dropped into a chair. When he had found what he was looking for, he sat down behind the desk and, without looking up, started to write. He was working on the report that he would have to give to the coroner that afternoon, in which he would have to describe Mrs. Kees's medical condition, the circumstances that had led to her euthanasia request, and the way in which it had been carried out. Occasionally, he paged through Mrs. Kees's case notes, read something, and then copied it into his report. When he was finished, he scooped all the papers together in an untidy bundle and hurried out the door, without once looking at me. He was nervous.

I got up and went to stand in the doorway so that I would have a view of the whole corridor. A woman in a green outfit with a matching cap passed. She disappeared into Mrs. Kees's room.

Inge, the head nurse, came out of the room. "That was the anesthetist," she said as she walked past. "They're inserting the intravenous line." A few minutes later, Inge returned up the corridor with Gerard, Elizabeth, and Karel. They all went into Mrs. Kees's room. I looked at my watch. Half an hour later, they emerged from the room, together with the woman in green. They had plastic carryall bags with Mrs. Kees's belongings. Mrs. Kees was already dead. The four of them walked down the corridor and through the swinging doors in silence. No one looked at me.

Then Mark came out of the room. As he hurried past, our eyes met. "I can't talk now," he said, his voice trembling with emotion, and he disappeared through the swinging doors.

THE CORONER

I sat down in the office to await the arrival of the coroner. At a quarter to three, Inge came to tell me that the coroner was at the reception desk and that Mark had been called. I went into the hall to wait for him. Fifteen minutes later he came out of the elevator. "He's here," Mark said nervously when he saw me. Together we walked to the reception desk. We introduced ourselves, and Mark explained briefly what I was doing. We went into the doctor's office. Once we were seated, Mark summarized the course of Mrs. Kees's illness, the circumstances that had led to her request for euthanasia, and his reasons for granting it. This lasted about a quarter of an hour. While Mark was talking, the coroner filled in a form. He noted Mark's name, address, medical specialization, and the details of Mrs. Kees's illness. He asked, in a dry, monotone voice, whether Mark had obtained a second opinion and whether he could have a photocopy of Mark's report and Mrs. Kees's euthanasia declaration. Mark Hansen went to make the photocopies. The whole discussion had lasted twenty minutes.

When Mark had gone, the coroner asked me about my research. He wanted to know whether I had spoken to Mrs. Kees and what I thought of the whole affair. He made notes.

THE ANESTHETIST

Exactly seven weeks after the death of Mrs. Kees, I had an interview with the anesthetist, Mieke Van der Ven, about another patient. At the end, I asked her about Mrs. Kees.

"I was only involved in her case for a very short time," she said. "Mark asked me to talk to her. Actually, it was a double request: he wanted to know whether she was fit enough for the operation, and he wanted my opinion on her euthanasia request. I approved the operation—her condition was good enough for that—and I spoke to her about euthanasia. That's when her fear of becoming comatose during the operation emerged. I tried to comfort her and told her that if we know that someone is terminally ill and can't communicate, we won't go on endlessly keeping them alive. And I asked her—Bang!—just like that, what she thought about euthanasia. That's when she told me the story of her husband. Do you know that story?"

I nodded.

"Yes? That he had lung cancer and wanted to put an end to it and that it turned out not to be so easy?"

I nodded again.

"She experienced that as very traumatic. And she didn't want that to happen to her. That's why she wanted to have everything arranged in time. Well, she had her operation, and, of course, it turned out to be hopeless: she was completely full of tumor. They then tried palliative treatment so that she could at least eat and drink and perhaps go home. But that didn't work. Her condition deteriorated rapidly, very rapidly. If she drank something, she vomited it straight out again. She was nauseous, felt rotten, and suffered increasing pain. Then I went to see her for the second time. . . . " She hesitated. "In the case notes, I wrote something like, 'Does she want to or doesn't she?'"

"I saw that," I said.

"Yes, at that time, she wasn't in such a bad condition as she was when she died. At the time I wrote that, she thought, 'I want to put an end to this, but, on the other hand, I can manage like this for a while as well.' That's the story she presented to me, anyway, and I wasn't sure what to make of it. I could understand her euthanasia request: increasing pain, no longer able to eat or drink, constantly nauseous and retching, feeling herself gradually slipping away. . . . And then in the background the nagging fear, 'What will they do with me if it gets so bad that I can't make my will clear anymore?'

"So she wanted to put an end to it before it got that far. But then she immediately added, 'But I'm okay for the moment.' So then I thought, 'Does she want to or doesn't she?' What I mean is, I had the impression that she *did* want to, but *not yet*.

"So then an independent doctor saw her to evaluate her request, and he confirmed that her suffering was unbearable and her request serious. The psychologist also went to see her. Then I received the message, 'Mrs. Kees has now said her good-byes and we have arranged a date.' It was the end of the week, and the date they had arranged was the following Wednesday. I went to see her for the third time, and I made definite arrangements with her for the Wednesday: who was going to be present, had she made all her own arrangements, was there anyone she still wanted to see, and did she really want to go ahead with it? It was a short discussion, but very intensive. I had the feeling that she was now really ready. And she was.

"On the Wednesday, I brought along all that was needed because we had agreed to do it quickly, which is what she wanted. Mark was there, and her son, daughter, and son-in-law. I asked her whether she still wanted to go ahead. She said, 'Everything is ready.' Well, I connected everything and in twenty-five minutes she was dead. It all happens very quickly."

"What did you give her?" I asked.

"You have to make sure that they fall asleep quickly, that they don't feel anything," she said. "So you give them an overdose of sedatives and painkillers. And then to be on the safe side, you always add a muscle relaxant. And if their condition is as bad as hers, then it all happens very quickly."

"I understand that there are different opinions here in the hospital about how to go about it. There are those who think that it should be done quickly and those who prefer to do it slowly by gradually increasing the morphine because they don't want the patient to die 'on the needle.' What do you think?"

"That depends on what the patient wants. I think that the patient should have a say, and I always ask them how they want it done. And the strange thing is that they almost always say, they want it to be quick—'Choek!'" She made a chopping motion with her hand. "I call it the guillotine method because they fall asleep and half an hour later they're dead. Patients say they want to do it like that because they want quick release from their own suffering, but they also don't want to drag things out for the friends and relatives. I try to empathize and do what they want, but, if I'm completely honest, I think it's *so unnatural* to die like that. I think—and maybe that's very

Calvinistic of me, but then we Dutch are imbued with Calvinism—that it's good for the friends and relatives if the patient dies slowly and gradually and that it's not such a bad thing if it takes a few hours. That gives them time to talk to, and about, the patient, to say good-bye properly, to recall experiences, to cry together—in short, to experience part of the mourning process at the bedside of the dying patient. These people miss that, and I'm not so sure whether that's a good thing. You can easily say, 'I've already said good-bye to my mother or father,' but when it actually happens, it's still a big shock. Of course, there are a lot of people who die in car accidents, and then [relatives] also have to cope with sudden death. But here the relatives have already been exposed to terminal illness, and they are already partly involved in the process of mourning, and then, Boom!, it's suddenly terminated, artificially.

"The relatives always thank me, happy that it was all so clean and fast, that the suffering of their loved one has finally come to an end. When the patient is asleep and in the final stage, I always try to get them to talk about the patient. It doesn't always work, though. When you have twenty of them sitting in the room like that, all silent, it's so horribly *unnatural.*

"And that applies to the doctors as well, particularly the junior doctors, who are so directly involved with the patient. They always find situations like that difficult. They don't sleep for nights afterward. For them, it's also part of a process of mourning, and if it's all much slower, much more natural, and those involved can laugh a bit and cry a bit, express their emotions, instead of sitting there in silence and repressing it, then it makes it a lot easier for everyone."

THE EUTHANASIA REQUEST

Mrs. Kees's euthanasia request developed out of a convergence of various factors. The basis was, of course, her terminal illness: the increasing pain, the continual retching, and the hopeless prognosis. The doctors had given her a couple of weeks at most to live, weeks of unbearable pain or increasing drowsiness.

Mrs. Kees had taken care of her mother, who had also died of stomach cancer, and she had been able to anticipate her own diagnosis and prognosis. But the death of her husband, of lung cancer five years earlier, was perhaps the most important factor. They had signed euthanasia declarations together, but she had seen him deteriorate and suffer because the GP refused to consider euthanasia; he felt that they had raised the issue too late. Both her children and her son-in-law had euthanasia declarations.

Mrs. Kees's personality and those of her children, as well as their mutual relationships, were also important, as was the fact that there were not many of them: the more relatives involved, the more likely are conflicts and differences of opinion. Mrs. Kees was sober minded and pragmatic. She knew exactly what she did and did not want. What she did not want was to suffer unnecessary pain or to become so drowsy that she could not decide for herself what was going to happen to her. Mrs. Kees had never been religious, so religious prohibitions against euthanasia played no role. Her children were also rational and pragmatic regarding questions of life and death: "Why wait, when you are going to die anyway?" her daughter, Elizabeth, had asked herself. Gerard, her son, told me that he had said good-bye to his mother emotionally a long time ago. Mrs. Kees, her two children, and her son-in-law remained calm and composed right to the end. I never saw tears, never heard anyone complain or curse fate. Their composure was not forced either. They did not give the impression that they were holding back or repressing their emotions. One hour before the euthanasia, Karel, the son-in-law, could greet me with a relaxed smile and Elizabeth and Gerard could wave and laugh.

I had expected things to be different. I also later experienced very different reactions to similar situations. A few days later, for example, I met another family of almost the same composition. The mother, who was the same age as Mrs. Kees, also had a terminal stomach cancer. Her sister had died a few years earlier of the same illness. Together with Gerrit Knol, another junior doctor, I attended the "bad news interview." The patient had been wheeled into the lounge, and her relatives sat claustrophobically around her. The daughter and son-in-law were sitting on the bed. The daughter was holding her mother's hand. The son sat in a chair on the other side of the bed and held her other hand. The grandmother sat at the foot of the bed. They were all tense, and no one could sit still.

"Well," Gerrit began, "I've got bad news . . . " He did not get any further. The daughter jumped up and screamed hysterically, "She's got *it!* she's got *it!* Goddamn, I knew it! What's she done to deserve this?" and rushed out of the door, kicking the cupboard as she left. The grandmother was rocking back and forth in her chair, moaning loudly, "Oh no, oh no, oh no." The son had leaned forward, and as tears rolled down his cheeks, he asked Gerrit, "Why, goddamn it, why? First her sister and now her. Is that fair?"

The woman died a few weeks later, without euthanasia ever being mentioned. It seemed as though those involved did not have the time to even think of it: they were all too busy with their emotions and the business of saying good-bye. According to the anesthetist, the Kees family was perhaps too rational: more emotion, even more suffering, would help the process of mourning, she said. Perhaps, but whatever the case, it is clear that the rational attitude of Mrs. Kees and her children, and the relative lack of emotion, contributed to the development and the fulfillment of her euthanasia request.

THE PARTICIPANTS

A patient and his or her relatives may be justified in requesting euthanasia, but if the doctor involved refuses to cooperate, then euthanasia cannot take place. This is clear in the case of Mrs. Kees's husband and the GP. In addition to all the personal factors that formed the background of Mrs. Kees's euthanasia request, the willingness of the various doctors and nurses who were involved, their personalities, their relationships with the patient and with each other, also played a role in the development and fulfillment of Mrs. Kees's request.

Mark Hansen was receptive to euthanasia requests and was prepared to discuss them with patients. He knew Mrs. Kees well and had a good relationship with her. Dr. Van Ham, who was officially in charge, was opposed to euthanasia but kept in the background. With Dr. Van Ham excluded from the decision-making process and support from the gastroenterologist, the anesthetist, the psychologist, and the nurses (who were all receptive to euthanasia requests), sufficient consensus existed to grant Mrs. Kees's request.

The harmonious situation on the internal ward was also favorable. The relationship between the doctor involved and the nurses was good, Mrs. Kees was popular (the nurses had had her brought back to their ward after her operation rather than letting her go to the surgical ward), and the nurses all supported her euthanasia request. So, given the patient's condition, her euthanasia request, the harmonious social environment, and the willingness of the staff to help her, the way was clear for the actual implementation.

DID SHE REALLY WANT TO DIE?

One question remains to be considered: did Mrs. Kees really want euthanasia? After all, doubts did surface along the way. "Does she want to or doesn't she?" the anesthetist had asked rhetorically in Mrs. Kees's case notes. Inge Fransen, the head nurse, also sometimes seemed to question Mrs. Kees's request. When she asked Mrs. Kees whether she had second thoughts, the latter had answered, "On the one hand, I do because I want to live, though only if I can be healthy. But whether it happens today or tomorrow, I'm going to die anyway, so then it's better to do it my way." Gerard's remark that it was "rather absurd" that his mother had decided to fix a date when she was in a "relatively bearable condition" could also be interpreted as doubt about the genuineness of her request.

These expressions of doubt can also be interpreted as part of a process in which all those involved had to adjust to what was happening. Indeed, it would have been strange if no one had expressed doubts or questioned Mrs. Kees's request. Of course, Mrs. Kees did not want to die. She would have liked to live, but her illness, her rapidly deteriorating condition, and the hopeless prognosis made this impossible, and in combination with the strong personality of a woman who wanted to have everything under her own control, the outcome was her euthanasia request. The doctors, however, had to seriously consider every expression of doubt. Each time she seemed to hesitate, her resolve had to be checked. After reading the anesthetist's question in the file, Inge Fransen had confronted Mrs. Kees directly, but Mrs. Kees had reiterated that she wanted to stick to the Wednesday appointment. When she wrote her question, the anesthetist had the impression that Mrs. Kees wanted euthanasia, but not yet. Later, as the Wednesday approached, she became convinced that Mrs. Kees was now ready.

The final interpretation, as Wednesday approached, was that Mrs. Kees's request was consistent. Mark Hansen, who probably knew her best, said that she was very persistent: "She wants euthanasia at all costs," he told me. "I only mentioned Wednesday, but she's keeping me to it. She's looking forward to it." And when Dr. Nieuwenhuis had had a discussion with her, he concluded "That's someone who really wants euthanasia, and who's thought about it for a long time." She also confirmed that she was ready in a discussion with the psychologist, and when the anesthetist saw her for the third time, she was also convinced: "I had the feeling that she was now really ready. And she was."

The doubt expressed by some of the participants was related to the difficulty of accepting that an exact date and time had been agreed upon for Mrs. Kees to die. Inge was not sure that this was "such a good idea," Gerard thought it was "absurd," and Elizabeth found it "strange."

Everyone agreed that Mrs. Kees was a strong and independent woman who knew exactly what she wanted. Her son-in-law said that she thought that there had been enough talking and enough delays. And when Inge asked her whether she was pushing forward with the euthanasia because she did not want to cause any trouble for her children, she denied it outright. "I'm very egotistical," she had said. "What I want, I get." This attitude is confirmed throughout the story of her request and its implementation. It is only apparently contradicted by Mrs. Kees's telling Inge that she did not want to die at home because she did not want to burden her children. It is doubtful, however, whether Mrs. Kees would have wanted to die at home anyway, given the traumatic experience with her husband and her only very superficial contact with her GP.

THE RULES OF DUE CARE

At the time of the my research, the rules of due care, which physicians who carried out euthanasia had to abide by if they wanted to avoid prosecution, were as follows:

- The doctor involved must be convinced that the request is voluntary and well considered.

- The patient should experience an enduring longing to die.
- The patient's suffering must be unbearable.
- The doctor must consult a colleague, preferably one who is not involved in the treatment of the patient.
- There must be a detailed written report containing the patient's case history, how the rules of due care were fulfilled, and the method used.
- Although not one of the rules of due care, it was assumed that the doctor would not fill in a natural cause of death on the death certificate and that he or she would report it as a case of euthanasia to the coroner.

Although Mrs. Kees had not initially directed her request for euthanasia to Mark Hansen, the attending physician, he was convinced that her request was voluntary and well considered. This interpretation was confirmed by all the other participants: her son and daughter; Dr. Nieuwenhuis, who had been consulted for a second opinion; the anesthetist; the nurses; and the psychologist. The specialist in charge, Dr. Van Ham, was opposed to euthanasia on religious grounds, but he did not interfere.

Given Mrs. Kees's condition and prognosis, all participants were convinced that her suffering was unbearable, and given her case history and the experience of her husband's illness, they were also convinced that she had an enduring longing to die.

Dr. Hansen had consulted a colleague who was not involved in Mrs. Kees's treatment (Dr. Nieuwenhuis) and had also involved the psychologist, the anesthetist, and the nursing staff in his decision.

He wrote a detailed report that he handed over, together with Mrs. Kees's euthanasia declaration and photocopies of relevant sections from the case notes, to the coroner.

He wrote "euthanasia" in on the death certificate and immediately reported the death as such to the coroner. This was euthanasia according to the rules, and, as a result, even though euthanasia was still a punishable offense under Article 293, no case was brought against Mark Hansen.

ON THE ROLE OF THE RESEARCHER ONCE MORE

Mrs. Kees's death was my initiation into, simultaneously, the hospital, the decision-making process relating to euthanasia, and the world of the dying patient. In many ways, Mrs. Kees resembled David in the previous chapter: they were both well aware of their situation, sober minded, and determined to have everything under their own control, right up until the end.

My role, however, was completely different. David was one of the last patients in whose death I was involved; Mrs. Kees was the first. With David I had spoken often, and with Mrs. Kees, not at all. Mrs. Kees had been willing to talk to me but could not because of an attack of retching. The next day she did not want to talk anymore. I had mixed feelings about this at the time. On the one hand, I wanted to talk to her because I had to find out how she had come to her decision, but, on the other hand, I did not want to talk to her, partly because I was not sure what questions would be acceptable to a terminally ill patient and partly because I found it embarrassingly selfish to occupy her last moments for the sake of my research.

In the course of my research, I had discussions with many terminal patients and their relatives. Sometimes I visited them at home. I learned how to assess patients and their situations: for some of them, death was a taboo subject, and we talked of football and television programs, whereas others sought me out in the hospital or phoned me at home in the evening to talk about death. The doubt about what I could acceptably ask and what I couldn't ask soon disappeared. The discomfort about my intrusion into their final moments remained but was mitigated by the discovery that some patients valued their discussions with me. I acquired a therapeutic role and, thus, a certain degree of legitimacy.

Chapter 3

Where the Responsibility Lies

MRS. VAN NELLE

After I had spent a number of weeks in the gastroenterology unit, Dr. Nieuwenhuis went on leave and I transferred my activities to pulmonology. Dr. Glas, one of the pulmonologists who had agreed to assist me in my research, had just returned from vacation, and I accompanied him to see one of his patients, Mrs. Van Nelle. We found her sitting on a sofa in the hall, smoking a cigarette. Dr. Glas asked her how she felt. She sighed deeply. "I just *can't* go on like this, you know," she said, looking up at him with an almost theatrical expression of suffering. "I've had enough. I don't want to go on like this." Her tone was slightly aggressive.

"I want to send you home," Dr. Glas said, in a friendly voice, "so that you can calm down in your own surroundings." I later heard that she had a long-running conflict with the nurses.

"But you *know* that's impossible." She sighed a few times, dramatically.

"In that, case we'll just have to keep you here in the hospital for the time being," Dr. Glas said.

"No! I can't go home, but I can't stay here either. I'm in pain and I don't want to go on," she complained.

Mrs. Van Nelle was fifty-five years old. She had a long and complicated medical history and was well known in the hospital. She frequently attended Dr. Glas's outpatient clinic because of her chronic bronchitis and emphysema. Both her mother and sister had died of cancer in their fifties, and Mrs. Van Nelle had lived in fear of the disease for years. She had had all kinds of illnesses, operations, and complications—her case history read like a textbook of internal medicine—but she was nonetheless thankful that she had been spared the ultimate horror of cancer.

That is, until a routine checkup in the autumn of 1990 revealed a tumor in her right lung. In the year following this diagnosis, she was admitted to the pulmonology ward on a number of occasions because of shortness of breath. A year later, in the autumn of 1991, she was admitted to the neurology ward because of persistent backache. Examination revealed spinal metastases. The pain in her back gradually became more intense, and in April 1992, she was again admitted for the placing of an epidural catheter to improve the administration of morphine. In May she reported attacks of asphyxia and was admitted to the pulmonology ward again. When the doctors could find no explanation, she was discharged and arrangements were made for her to receive oxygen at home. In the following weeks, she phoned Dr. Glas frequently to say that she was short of breath and wanted to be readmitted to hospital. Medicine prescribed through the outpatient clinic was not working, she said. Meanwhile, Mr. Van Nelle had informed the hospital that the situation at home was untenable. Home care was mobilized, but the Van Nelles were still not satisfied.

Mrs. Van Nelle was finally admitted for a checkup in August and reported weakness in her legs. This increased during her stay in hospital, and after a few days she could hardly walk at all. It was at that time that I first came across the word euthanasia in the nursing records:

> The patient has mentioned euthanasia. She was told to wait for Dr. Glas to come back from leave and discuss it with him.

Mrs. Van Nelle did not use the word euthanasia herself. She said that she had had enough and did not want to go on like this. In the following days, she complained frequently about backache. She hardly slept at night and summoned the nurses to her bedside regularly with the emergency bell. She said that she felt more miserable by the hour and was beginning to lose her grip on things. She became edematous and her legs and face puffed up. She started to produce bloody stools. She told one of the nurses that she did not want to go home anymore because she was worried that she would not be cared for properly. She was short of breath, and walking was increasingly difficult because of the pain in her back.

At the beginning of September, just before Dr. Glas's return from vacation, one of the nurses noted the following:

> Mrs. Van Nelle has repeated her euthanasia request. She is angry that "they" do not think that she is ready for it. The anesthetist agrees that she isn't ready. Mrs. Van Nelle says she doesn't want to talk about it. "The doctor must do it without me knowing," she says. "Secretly, through an intravenous drip or something like that." She also wants to go home, but her family can't cope. She says that the home care people don't do a thing. When I asked her why she always agrees to be treated (the radiation therapy, for example), she says that the doctors always "con" her into it with their enthusiasm. She even says that it's "criminal" for them to keep her alive by such devious means.

SHE WANTS EUTHANASIA, BUT SHE IS AFRAID TO TAKE THE RESPONSIBILITY

On September 12, 1992, Mrs. Van Nelle was transferred from the pulmonology to the neurology ward—officially, because the neurologist was going to try to improve her mobility but, in fact, because the nurses in pulmonology needed a break from all the conflicts and tension that Mrs. Van Nelle tended to bring in her wake. On the neurology ward, trouble started almost immediately. On the very first evening after her transfer, Mrs. Van Nelle proclaimed loudly that she was dying of cancer and that the doctors could do nothing to alleviate her suffering. This caused some consternation, as Mrs. Van Nelle was now sharing a room with five other cancer patients. A private room was hastily organized and Mrs. Van Nelle was moved. From her new room, she made much use of the emergency bell to summon nurses to her bedside to complain about pain and shortness of breath and to emphasize that she did not want to go on.

A note in the nursing report, dated a few days later, read as follows:

> The patient is becoming despondent. Worries about her future. Keeps mentioning euthanasia, but she's not mentally ready for it yet. Need to liaise with psychologist. Demands a lot of attention. Pain alleviation is very difficult and with varying results!

The next day, Mrs. Van Nelle told the psychologist that she thought that her pain could not be adequately managed. She said that she now accepted that she was going to die but was afraid of the moment of death. She said that she was not getting the support she needed as she approached death. And, she emphasized, she did not want to go to a nursing home. When the psychologist spoke to Mr. Van Nelle later the same day, he said that he and his daughter could no longer cope at home and that a nursing home was the only alternative. He thought that the question of euthanasia should remain open as a possibility but admitted to doubting the consistency of his wife's request. He said that her behavior and her moods had changed during the course of her illness. He wanted the psychologist to talk to her so that he would not have to tell her that she must go to a nursing home.

During the following days, the problems continued. Mrs. Van Nelle claimed that her morphine pump was not working properly and that she was suffering unnecessary pain. She made extensive use of the emergency bell and complained bitterly if the nurses did not respond immediately. She phoned her husband in the middle of the night and demanded that he come to the hospital. She had a telephone installed next to her bed and attached a large sign to it reading, PRIVATE—MRS. VAN NELLE.

During this period, the Van Nelles submitted a number of complaints to the hospital director concerning what they saw as the poor coordination among the different specialists who were involved in Mrs. Van Nelle's treatment. It was also during this period that I first met Mrs. Van Nelle, in the hall, when I was accompanying Dr. Glas on his rounds just after he had returned from vacation.

In the meantime, the neurologist told the psychologist that he had decided that he could not grant Mrs. Van Nelle's euthanasia request. He was scared that Mr. Van Nelle and his daughter might change their minds afterward and submit a complaint. "I must admit that the thought had also crossed my mind," the psychologist answered.

On September 23, a meeting took place between the neurologist, the junior neurology doctor, the anesthetist, and the Van Nelles. The neurologist explained to Mrs. Van Nelle that she could not remain in the hospital indefinitely, that rehabilitation was not an option, and that she would probably have to choose between intensive home care and a nursing home.

"You'll have to decide that for yourselves and inform us what your decision is later this week," the neurologist said.

"Oh no!" Mrs. Van Nelle exclaimed. "*I'm* not participating in that. I'm not going to take sides. *They* must decide," she said, indicating her husband and daughter with a nod of her head.

During that week, the psychologist had a number of discussions with the Van Nelles. When she told me about them, the psychologist said, "My plan was to get her to tell me what she thought of the matter. But all she said was, 'I can't take it anymore. What I really want is euthanasia, but I'm scared of the moment of death. So I want them to give me a jab without me knowing.' She kept expressing the problem like that. She simply laid her problem on the table—Bang!—just like that, and we had to find a solution for her. Then [Mr. Van Nelle] started about them being members of the Association [Association for Voluntary Euthanasia]. 'It's *your* decision, and nobody else can make it for you,' I told her. 'And only when you've made that decision can we discuss the method.' Her answer was that she couldn't go on, that she had *really* had enough. She started to cry and tell the whole old story once more. She went into a long litany of how she was suffering, how unbearable the nights were, and so on and so forth."

In her report, the psychologist wrote the following:

> She expresses a consistent and persistent wish for euthanasia but is afraid to take full responsibility for the decision herself. I told her that nobody can make that decision for her. She says that she would prefer to die in her sleep, without knowing. Her strength and resistance seem limited; her misery is overwhelming her. The willingness to struggle on seems to be absent. She admitted that her fear of death might be a cover for doubt about the decision. I

can't discover how she really feels. She expresses her feelings primarily through demanding solutions and helplessness and dissatisfaction. On the other hand, I must admit that I wouldn't want to change places with her. We mustn't expect the impossible of her.

On Friday, September 26, I was in Dr. Glas's office, waiting for him to finish writing a report, after which we were to go to see Mrs. Van Nelle. The door was open and Mieke Van der Ven, the anesthetist, passed. She caught sight of us and stopped.

"Yesssss," she said, with a long hiss of air as she leaned against the doorjamb. "She's a difficult woman. She has a lot of pent-up aggression against the clinical staff. In fact, the whole family has a lot of pent-up aggression against the hospital. She's continually expressing the desire for euthanasia, but she's too afraid to take the responsibility herself. I've got nothing against euthanasia, but I wouldn't fancy having problems with the relatives afterwards just because she didn't want to take the responsibility herself."

"I don't think it would be a good idea to let her die here in the hospital," Dr. Glas said. "I want to get her home so that she can calm down in a familiar environment. She's very difficult, and the nurses can't cope with her much longer. I've known her for years: she was always a difficult woman."

When we were on our way to see Mrs. Van Nelle, Dr. Glas told me that the anesthetist was responsible for Mrs. Van Nelle's pain medication. "She also plays a role in the implementation of euthanasia," he continued. "Actually, I'm not very happy with the way the anesthetists go about euthanasia. The patient literally dies on the needle. It's a question of giving a shot, counting to ten, and the patient is dead. The doctor also needs to experience some kind of a mourning process, and a quick, technical implementation doesn't make things easier. I prefer to let them go gradually with a morphine infusion. It's much more peaceful and less traumatic for all those involved. It's a much more natural way of dying."

When we entered Mrs. Van Nelle's room, Dr. Glas asked her how she was feeling. She sighed dramatically. "I've pressed the bell four times in the last five minutes and still no one has come." To demonstrate, she held up the remote control of the emergency bell and then let it drop onto the bed. "You see? They're making me wait on purpose, when they know I'm in pain." She looked up at Dr. Glas, and her eyebrows, which had been wrinkled into a frown, relaxed, and her indignant tone mellowed and became one of suffering and affliction. "And I *am* in so much pain, doctor," she said. "I really can't take it anymore."

"Yes," Dr. Glas said. "We can't go on like this. I'll have you transferred to my unit, and then we'll talk about increasing the morphine so that you *really* won't have any pain."

INCREASING THE MORPHINE

I arrived on the pulmonology ward on Monday morning to find Mrs. Van Nelle installed in a private room. She looked in much better spirits. "I'm *so* glad to be back," she said cheerfully. "And the nurses here are *so* good to me."

"Why did you change your mind about sending her home?" I asked Dr. Glas when he arrived on the ward.

"I was planning to," he said, "but it wasn't feasible. Now that she's here, I can increase the pain medication, and once she's calmed down, we can talk about how we can let her go to sleep peacefully because, as it is, the situation is hopeless."

"Why wasn't it possible to send her home?" I asked.

"The home care people couldn't get things organized at such short notice and . . . well, the Van Nelles have had enough conflicts with home care in the past as well. . . . Their GP also wasn't very enthusiastic. The idea is to give her high doses of morphine through an intravenous line—pain alleviation and nothing else. Whatever else we do simply decreases her quality of life. She's said good-bye to her family, and we're hoping for a respiratory suppression. We'd hoped that it would have happened spontaneously before now."

Later that day, I had an appointment with Marthe Diepen, the psychologist. Dr. Glas came along to inform her that he had transferred Mrs. Van Nelle to his unit.

"Why was she transferred from your unit to neurology in the first place anyway?" the psychologist asked. "You know how they think about these matters in neurology, namely, not at all."

"It happened during my leave because of problems with the nurses," Dr. Glas answered. "Now that she's back we can increase the morphine, perhaps with Valium."

"The anesthetists are not so happy with that method," said the psychologist.

"Yes, if you give her a muscle relaxant, she'll be gone in no time," said Dr. Glas.

"Then it's not going to be euthanasia?" she asked.

"*Only* symptom alleviation," Dr. Glas emphasized. "It's going to be a natural dying process."

After my discussion with the psychologist, I walked back to the ward, where Dr. Glas was scheduled to have a discussion with the Van Nelles. I waited for him in the corridor, and we entered Mrs. Van Nelle's room together. She was in bed, and her husband and daughter were present.

"I can't take this anymore," she said, as soon as she saw Dr. Glas. "I feel pain everywhere, and the medicine isn't helping, and I'm suffocating. Life has become a torture. I don't see why I'm being made to suffer like this." She rolled her eyes and looked up at the ceiling for a few seconds.

"That's exactly what I came to talk to you about," Dr. Glas said. "What we're going to do about that pain. I want to increase the morphine through an intravenous line, and then you'll probably go to sleep peacefully."

"I'm so scared of the moment of death, of the unknown," she said, as she looked straight at Dr. Glas, her lips white.

"There's no need to worry about that. Dying will just be the same as going to sleep. When we increase the morphine, you'll fall into a deep sleep. It'll be just as though you were tired and longing for sleep. Once you're asleep, you'll drop into a CO_2 [carbon dioxide] narcosis, and the brain functions will gradually close down, starting with the higher functions, until only the stem and the basic functions are still working— "

"But what if I suffocate . . . ?"

"No, you won't suffocate. You won't notice a thing. I'm going to get the anesthetist to install an intravenous line so that we can start increasing the morphine. And as a result of that, you'll go to sleep peacefully."

"But I'm so scared that I'll wake up."

"No, you won't wake up. If there's any chance of that I'll give you a sedative."

Mrs. Van Nelle breathed a sigh of relief and laid her head back on her pillows. Mr. Van Nelle nodded in agreement. That evening one of the nurses wrote the following:

> Euthanasia discussion has taken place. The dying process will be hastened during the coming days. Exactly how and when, Mrs. Van Nelle couldn't tell me. The anesthetist and the psychologist will be involved. From tomorrow, Mr. Van Nelle will be sleeping here together with his wife. Both are relieved.

The next morning at half past eight, I went to see Mrs. Van Nelle. She said that she hadn't slept well because of the pain, but she hadn't wanted to use the emergency bell because the nurses were busy enough as it was. She said that she was happy that she was finally going to be delivered from her suffering.

After leaving Mrs. Van Nelle, I went into the doctor's office, where I heard the ward doctor speaking to the anesthetist on the phone. He was asking her whether she could come to install an intravenous line for Mrs. Van Nelle. This she did a few minutes later, leaving again as quickly as she had arrived. Not long after that, Mrs. Van Nelle went to the hospital library and borrowed three books. She then spent the rest of the morning reading quietly in her room. Her husband and daughter were due later.

At eleven I went to see her again. Now she was lying on her bed. She was in a good mood and chattered away amicably, until the physiotherapist came in. "I don't want *that* anymore," she said distastefully. "It's painful and requires too much effort. And, in any case, it's unnecessary because I gather that I'm not going to be around much longer. So let's not bother."

The physiotherapist, used to such snubs, wondered whether Mrs. Van Nelle might like to have some light exercise, but she was not interested in that either. "Then why don't you just lie right there and I'll massage your legs for you," the physiotherapist suggested. Mrs. Van Nelle thought that that was a good idea, and I left them to it.

At one o'clock, Dr. Glas came onto the ward and told one of the nurses that it was time to start the morphine. Mrs. Van Nelle was in her room reading. She had been there since the physiotherapist left more than an hour earlier. Dr. Glas went into her room with one of the nurses, and me in his wake, and told her that they were going to start with the morphine.

"Things *are* moving rather quickly now, aren't they?" she asked, looking up from her book.

"Okay, we'll wait until you go to bed then. We don't want you dropping off in your chair, do we?" he said. Mrs. Van Nelle looked at him but said nothing.

Usually Mrs. Van Nelle went to bed after lunch because the pain in her back became unbearable if she was up for more than a few hours. Today, however, she did not want to go to bed, preferring to remain in her chair. When that became too painful, she got into bed but had her husband roll her out of the room and into the hall. At quarter past two, one of the junior doctors came into the doctor's office to pick up a file. "Are you waiting for *that?*" she said, indicating Mrs. Van Nelle's room with her head.

I nodded. "What do you think?"

"I don't want to get involved," she said. "I've just seen her in her bed in the hall, laughing and smoking. It's not at all clear what she really wants." She turned and left with the file under her arm.

At three, the ward doctor gave the student nurses a lecture about lung cancer. I joined them, and the discussion soon turned to Mrs. Van Nelle. The nurses were unhappy about the course of events. It had been agreed that a couple of nurses would be present at the last meeting between Dr. Glas and the Van Nelles, but when Dr. Glas arrived on the ward, he went straight to Mrs. Van Nelle's room without informing the nurses. When they realized Dr. Glas was already there, they hurried to Mrs. Van Nelle's room, only to find the door closed, and they did not dare to go in. As a result, no nurse representative was present to hear what had been agreed. They were irritated that they had not been involved in the discussion about euthanasia. They had heard rumors about euthanasia but were not sure exactly what was going on. They felt they had a right to know, as they were the ones looking after Mrs. Van Nelle. They didn't want to come to work one day and discover that their patient had been euthanized.

When I returned to the doctor's office at half past four, I noticed that Mrs. Van Nelle was back in her room. Through the open door I could see Mieke Van der Ven, the anesthetist, sitting on the edge of the bed. A few minutes later she came into the office.

"I've just been to say good-bye," she said to the ward doctor. "I'm not satisfied with the way things are going. I'm unhappy about the decision to use morphine."

"That's Dr. Glas's way of doing things," he said with a shrug. "I suspected that you were dissatisfied because you didn't write much in the report."

She nodded. "I'll keep what I really think to myself."

At quarter to five, Dr. Glas went to see Mrs. Van Nelle to discuss what to do next. I followed. Mrs. Van Nelle was in bed, propped up with large pillows. "Can't we start off with a smaller dosage?" she asked, before Dr. Glas had a chance to say anything.

"That's what I've come to discuss with you," he said. "You're the one who ultimately has to decide. But if you want to be really free of pain, then we're going to have to increase the morphine as we agreed earlier."

"But can you guarantee that I won't get drowsy?"

"No. I can't guarantee that, but the point is to make sure you're not in pain."

"The pain isn't important. I've had so much pain, a bit more won't do any harm. I want to be clearheaded up to the end. I only want you to increase the morphine if you guarantee that I'm not going to become drowsy."

"But I can't."

"Okay, then I don't want the morphine. I must stay clearheaded till the end. And I want to wait until my daughter arrives before we discuss [this] further." She was now in a more militant mood and started to complain about the neurologist.

After going on for a while, she looked at Dr. Glas sentimentally. "But I'm *very* grateful to be back here with you," she said.

As a result of this meeting, Dr. Glas informed the nurse in charge to keep the morphine on hold and only start it if Mrs. Van Nelle requested it herself. By seven o'clock, Mrs. Van Nelle was again in pain and the morphine was started. Fifteen minutes later, she rang the emergency bell and said she wanted the morphine turned off because she was feeling drowsy. She spent the rest of the evening smoking in bed.

Smoking was not allowed, but Mrs. Van Nelle was a difficult woman and took no notice of the rules. The nurses, who all smoked themselves during breaks—much to Dr. Glas's anger—would have had a serious fight on their hands if they had tried to stop her. She considered smoking to be one of the few pleasures left to her in her final days, as did many other terminally ill lung cancer patients.

Mr. Van Nelle was also present and had a bed of his own in his wife's room.

Just after midnight, Mrs. Van Nelle rang the bell again. She was in pain and short of breath. She wanted to start the morphine again. The nurse started the infusion, and half an hour later, Mrs. Van Nelle was sleeping peacefully.

When I arrived on the ward the next morning at half past eight, Dr. Glas had already been to see Mrs. Van Nelle. He told me that she was in a deep sleep and did not react when spoken to. Given the condition of her lungs, he expected her to die that day.

At half past ten, I went to see her myself. Her head was bent back over the pillow and her chin pointed up at the ceiling. Her mouth was open, and without her dentures for support her lips and cheeks had sagged inward. Her face was pale. Occasionally a shudder passed through her body and there was a gurgling sound in her throat.

Fifteen minutes later, Dr. Glas came onto the ward to inform the nurses that they could increase the morphine further and give her Dormicum, a sedative, if the need arose. We then went to Mrs. Van Nelle's room, where her husband had just relieved her daughter at the bedside. Dr. Glas went up to Mrs. Van Nelle and looked at her closely.

"Don't worry about the noises," he said to Mr. Van Nelle. "The higher brain functions have already been shut down, and she's not conscious of anything. I'm going to increase the morphine, and then she will soon pass away."

"Please do, Doctor," said Mr. Van Nelle.

Mrs. Van Nelle died three quarters of an hour later. On the death certificate, Dr. Glas filled in "respiratory insufficiency" as the cause of death.

WAS SHE SUFFERING UNBEARABLY?

Some weeks after Mrs. Van Nelle's death, the anesthetist told me that she had never really understood Mrs. Van Nelle's pain. "Her body didn't seem to confirm what she was telling us," she said. "She could tell you with a smile that she was suffering *unbearable* pain and that she couldn't *stand* it a moment longer. And then ten minutes later, you saw her sitting in the hall, chatting and laughing and eating French fries or smoking a cigarette, and not a sign of pain anywhere. So it was almost impossible to evaluate the treatment I was giving her. I still don't know to what extent it helped." This was echoed by other doctors as well.

Although the exact nature and extent of Mrs. Van Nelle's suffering was unclear, everyone was convinced that she *was* suffering. The consensus among medical staff in the hospital was that if a patient claimed to be in pain then they must assume that the patient *is* in pain, whether or not they could identify a clear physical source of that pain. Another issue was nonphysical. Here, I do not want to initiate a discussion of the nature of suffering and at what point it becomes unbearable, but it was clear that mental suffering also played a role in Mrs. Van Nelle's euthanasia request. At the time this study was carried out, mental suffering was not, in itself, officially recognized as a justification for granting a euthanasia request, but opinion in the Netherlands was shifting, and many doctors considered mental suffering, particularly when accompanied by an incurable physical illness, to be a sufficient condition for considering a euthanasia request. (Not long after Mrs. Van Nelle's death, the well-publicized *Chabot* case—in which a psychiatrist was acquitted after assisting the suicide of a woman who was depressive but had no physical illness—shifted Dutch jurisprudence further, confirming mental suffering per se as justifiable grounds for euthanasia.)

As a result, most of those involved accepted that Mrs. Van Nelle was suffering sufficiently to justify her euthanasia request. The questions remained: Was that request serious? Did Mrs. Van Nelle really want to die?

DID SHE REALLY WANT TO DIE?

Here, also, there was ambiguity. The anesthetist reported that Mrs. Van Nelle mentioned euthanasia every time she saw her, but either indirectly or qualified by the remark, "But I'm not ready for it yet."

"She kept saying that right up to the end," the anesthetist told me. "Which meant that, in spite of all the complaints, she didn't consider herself to be so sick that she could request euthanasia directly. But she *was* requesting it, only to deny it immediately after. And that's what I found so difficult. You had the impression that she wanted you to say, 'Okay, listen, you've got metastasized cancer, you've got worn-out lungs, you can't walk, you can't manage to take a bath by yourself, you can't do anything. In fact, you're in such a bad condition that you can ask for euthanasia.' *That's* what she wanted you to tell her every time you saw her. And if you did say it, then she immediately changed the subject. So you were never sure whether it was a real request or whether she just wanted confirmation that she was permitted to think about the possibility."

Even Mr. Van Nelle occasionally expressed doubt about the consistency of his wife's euthanasia request.

Her behavior was also ambiguous. When Dr. Glas agreed to increase the morphine through an intravenous line, he said that his primary aim was to alleviate her pain, although everyone, including Mrs. Van Nelle herself, knew that her death would be hastened by this. That was, after all, what she had been asking for. She seemed content with the arrangement, and after it had been made, she was calm and composed. She even refused physiotherapy because, as she put it, she was not "going to be around much longer." That morning, however, she borrowed three books from the library and spent the rest of the day diligently reading, when she must have known that, if all went according to plan, she would never get beyond the first couple of chapters at most.

Then, in the afternoon, when Dr. Glas came to inform her that it was time to start the morphine, she thought that things were "moving rather quickly." Dr. Glas said that they could wait until she went to bed, which she normally did straight after lunch, but that day she stayed up until well into the afternoon. When the pain in her back became too much and she finally had to go to bed, she got her husband to wheel her into the hall, where she spent the rest of the afternoon. When she finally returned to her room, she told Dr. Glas that she only wanted morphine if he could guarantee that it would not make her drowsy, even though she must have known that this was impossible. When the pain became unbearable, she asked for morphine, only to have it stopped again after fifteen minutes. Then she summoned the nurse in the middle of the night to start the morphine again, and she fell asleep and never woke up again.

This ambiguity was compounded by the fact that she was difficult. When she was admitted to a ward, she had arguments with the nurses and complaints from other patients multiplied. Mr. and Mrs. Van Nelle regularly submitted complaints to the hospital director about various members of the medical staff. She complained to one specialist about another, pit the nurses against the doctors, and fomented conflict between the hospital specialists and her GP. The various parties became annoyed with one another, while trying their best to empathize with Mrs. Van Nelle, despite the realization that she was setting them up. They did their best to explain her behavior and her complaints as a consequence of her illness and the pain she was suffering, and everyone thought that her euthanasia request was justified. But because she refused to explicitly take responsibility for the decision, they hesitated.

Although it was not entirely clear whether Mrs. Van Nelle *really* wanted to die, Dr. Glas nonetheless continued to increase the morphine until she did die. Afterward, when he had taken the burden for the decision upon himself, and all the tensions and fears had receded, a general consensus formed among most of those involved that Dr. Glas had interpreted Mrs. Van Nelle's request correctly and had been justified in his decision to help her:

The GP: "I'm glad that Glas delivered her from her suffering. Mr. Van Nelle told me that it was a very humane death. I don't know what Glas filled in on the death certificate as the cause of death, but if there's ever an investigation, then I'll support his decision fully. Her suffering was really unbearable and hopeless."

The junior neurologist: "She submitted complaints to the director for the most trivial things, and that is one of the reasons why we [the neurology unit] were so hesitant with regard to euthanasia; because before you know it, they'd have complained about that too. It was really good of Glas that he didn't just abandon her to a nursing home. He knew her well, of course, and was in a position to evaluate the situation."

The anesthetist: "I think that he did what she wanted. But I'm not sure she wanted it as quickly as that . . . she was dead twenty-four hours after the start of the treatment. And then he gave her a sedative in addition to the pain medication as well. Well, I suppose that's his responsibility. But I do think that by doing so he did her a big. . . . He took the decision out of her hands, when it should have been in her hands. He did that because he thought that she wanted him to, and I think that's beautiful. I assume that his conscience is clear. I think it is. I can understand why he did it. It's a kind of, well . . . fatherly authority, a responsibility that you take over from your child. It's a bit paternalistic, without too many of the negative connotations of the word. So I understand why he did it, but I think, I hope, that it gives him a few sleepless nights nonetheless."

Mr. Van Nelle: I never spoke to Mr. Van Nelle again, but two days after his wife's death, he sent Dr. Glas a card. On it he had written, "With sincere thanks for shortening my wife's suffering."

However, not everybody agreed with the dominant interpretation of events. Shortly after Mrs. Van Nelle's death, I had a discussion with Jan Smit, one of the nurses who had been involved in Mrs. Van Nelle's care.

"I really had the feeling that she was killed when she didn't want to die," he told me. "On the one hand, I think she was having a horrible time and that she had a horrible life; I'm convinced of that. But I'm also convinced that there was also some satisfaction and a few pleasant moments in that horrible life, even if it was only the pleasure of making other people angry. I think she thought that she was a burden on the nurses—and she was a burden—and that that's why she said she wanted to die. And they took her up on it, and, well, then she decided she didn't want to, but she had reached the point that she couldn't—at least that was my interpretation—say that she didn't want to. After that, they continued to increase the morphine, and she died. I really have the feeling that she was killed when, deep in her heart, she didn't want to go through with it. Maybe she only asked for the morphine to be turned on again with the intention of temporary relief, just to sleep for a few hours. But maybe I've got it all wrong."

DR. GLAS'S INTENTION

Everyone agreed that Dr. Glas had shortened Mrs. Van Nelle's life, and most of those involved thought that this was what she really wanted. But was it euthanasia? (I am referring to euthanasia as officially defined, not to the ambiguous individual definitions often employed in practice.) The problem here is that the same medication and means of administration can be used for both symptom alleviation *and* euthanasia. Because a patient might request euthanasia, and at the same time need a substantial increase in symptom alleviation, it is only the physician's motive that determines whether these actions constitute euthanasia or normal medical practice.

Van der Wal and Van der Maas (1996:41) distinguish three categories of intention in this context:

1. Not intending to hasten the patient's death, but taking into account the probability or the certainty that the patient's death would thereby be hastened
2. Having the express purpose of hastening the patient's death
3. Partially intending to hasten the patient's death

Taking the basic empirical actions described in the case of Mrs. Van Nelle (patient is terminally ill and suffering; patient requests euthanasia; the doctor increases the morphine; the patient's death is hastened; the doctor does not report his actions as euthanasia) and combining these with the three categories of intention, we get three different situations, each with a different official outcome and different legal consequences:

1. If Dr. Glas had increased the morphine with the *intention of alleviating pain and shortness of breath, with death as a concomitant but unintended consequence,* then, according to present Dutch policy, this would be seen as "normal medical practice," and Dr. Glas's actions would not be subject to further legal scrutiny.
2. If, however, he had carried out exactly the same actions with the *express purpose of accelerating Mrs. Van Nelle's death,* and these actions had been in response to a clear and consistent request from Mrs. Van Nelle, then his actions would be considered euthanasia by the authorities and subject to legal scrutiny, though he would not be prosecuted if he had kept to the rules of due care and not filled in a natural death on the death certificate.
3. If the situation had been exactly the same as in number 2, but Dr. Glas had *partially intended to hasten Mrs. Van Nelle's death,* then his actions would be subject to legal scrutiny, though he would not be prosecuted if he had kept to the rules of due care and not filled in a natural death on the death certificate.

In such situations, the doctor's intention determines the distinction between normal medical practice and euthanasia. It also determines whether he is likely to report his actions as euthanasia:

- If he only intends his actions as symptom alleviation, then he is not likely to report.
- If he has the express intention of hastening the patient's death, then if he doesn't report, he must have made a conscious decision not to.
- If he partially intends to hasten the patient's death, then whether he reports his actions as euthanasia depends on the extent to which he is aware of these different intentions, and whether he defines his actions and intentions in such a way that hastening the patient's death is the dominant intention.

The outcome (i.e., whether his actions are subject to the possibility of legal scrutiny) then depends on whether the doctor reports, which in turn depends on how he defines his own intentions.

These are ideal types: as Van der Wal and Van der Maas (1996) state, a doctor's intention is probably never *only* hastening death. Hastening death is always concomitant to alleviating suffering. The "express purpose" cases also will never only be that. There will also be some aspect of symptom alleviation. In addition, the boundaries between the different categories are fluid.

Assuming that Mrs. Van Nelle did have a clear and consistent request (if she did not, then the situation becomes more complex), then Dr. Glas's intentions are crucial in determining whether his actions constituted symptom alleviation or euthanasia. These actions would seem to fall into the third category (partially intending to hasten the patient's death), but some ambiguities do exist. To me, Dr. Glas said, "The idea is to give her high doses of morphine through an intravenous line—pain alleviation and nothing else. Whatever else we do simply decreases her quality of life. She's said good-bye to her family, and we're hoping for a respiratory suppression. We'd hoped that it would have happened spontaneously before now."

Here, Dr. Glas seems to say that the increased morphine is intended only for symptom alleviation. In the first sentence, "and nothing else" seems to refer to euthanasia (i.e., it's going to be symptom alleviation and not euthanasia). The second sentence, however, suggests that he is not making a distinction between symptom alleviation and euthanasia but rather between symptom alleviation and other medication (i.e., medication that is keeping her alive). This leaves open the possibility that Dr. Glas is referring to euthanasia and not exclusively to symptom alleviation.

But shortly afterward, when the psychologist asked explicitly whether Mrs. Van Nelle's death was to be euthansia, Dr. Glas replied that he was only going to provide symptom alleviation and that it would be a natural dying process.

Then again, other statements seem to contradict this intention. For example, when Mrs. Van Nelle had been transferred to the pulmonology ward, Dr. Glas explained to me, "Now that she's [in my unit] I can increase the pain medication, and once she's calmed down, we can talk about how we can let her go to sleep peacefully because, as it is, the situation is hopeless." The Dutch word *inslapen* means "to go to sleep," but it also means "to die." Dr. Glas also used this expression when speaking to Mrs. Van Nelle: "That's exactly what I came to talk to you about," Dr. Glas said to her. "What we're going to do about that pain. I want to increase the morphine through an intravenous line, and then you'll probably go to sleep peacefully." This interpretation is confirmed when Mrs. Van Nelle answers by saying, "I'm so scared of the moment of death . . . , " and Dr. Glas then goes on to describe the dying process.

When the psychologist asked whether Mrs. Van Nelle's death was going to be euthanasia, Dr. Glas denied this explicitly, but the nurses continued to talk of "arrangements for euthanasia." After the previous discussion about "going to sleep," the nurses noted in their report, "Euthanasia discussion has taken place." Dr. Glas must have read this report, and if he was not intending his actions to be euthanasia, why did he not contradict this statement?

Intentions may change from one situation to another, and it is possible that symptom alleviation was uppermost in Dr. Glas's mind when he was talking to the psychologist, but that this was replaced by other intentions when he was confronted by Mrs. Van Nelle's requests and her apparent suffering. His intentions might also have been equivocal: perhaps he was not entirely sure whether he wanted to grant her request.

One may still wonder, however, was it necessary in the context of sheer symptom alleviation, to keep increasing the morphine once Mrs. Van Nelle was asleep? Should Dr. Glas have waited, as Jan Smit suggested, until she woke up again before giving her the next dose? Perhaps, but would he then have delivered her from her pain as he had promised her he would?

Cases such as that of Mrs. Van Nelle show how difficult it is to determine what "taking into account the probability or the certainty that the patient's death would thereby be hastened" and "the partly intended hastening of the patient's death" mean in practice (Van der Wal and Van der Maas, 1996: 77, 92).

ASSUMING RESPONSIBILITY

In addition to the official guidelines that govern when the granting of a euthanasia request is justified (unbearable suffering, clear and consistent request, etc.), other implicit "rules" are utilized by doctors when confronted with a request for euthanasia. Before a doctor will seriously consider granting a patient's request for euthanasia, the patient must be seen as taking ultimate responsibility for the decision. Here, I am not simply generalizing from a single case, but from the observation of many euthanasia decisions throughout the study. Of course, Mrs. Van Nelle was not typical, and hers was, indeed, a problematic case because she refused to take the responsibility, but it is *because* of this that the "rule" emerges all the more clearly. In a case such as that of Mrs. Kees (see Chapter 2), in which the patient so unequivocally accepted full responsibility for the decision, this rule remains hidden and implicit.

What also emerges is that, if the patient is thought to have a legitimate request but is seen as being incapable of explicitly taking responsibility for the decision, it may, under certain circumstances, be considered acceptable for the doctor to assume this burden, an action that is, in the words of the anesthetist, "a bit paternalistic, without too many of the negative connotations of the word." Here, I assume that Mrs. Van Nelle did have a real desire to die, even though, as some claimed, she might not have wanted to die *that* quickly. When the doctor makes such a decision, support of colleagues, however implicit, is essential. The doctor in question needs to have sufficient skills to interpret the seriousness of the patient's request *and* to gauge, from indirect and implicit signs, the extent to which his or her colleagues will consider the assumption of a paternalistic authority to be legitimate *post facto*.

In the case of Mrs. Van Nelle, this assumption of responsibility was further exacerbated by the fact that she was so difficult and by the possibility of an official complaint from Mr. Van Nelle. It is easier to grant the request of a "nice" patient. "When you start to play God," the psychologist once said, "there's the danger that, with someone like Mrs. Van Nelle, you're going to think, 'I don't like the way she put that so I'm not going to grant her request.' Whereas with someone like Mrs. Kees, who was so balanced and heroic to the end, and who made it a lot easier for us, we think, 'For her, we'll do it.' Most people are not like that, but we have to listen to them as well. . . . "

Chapter 4

The Line Between Euthanasia and Symptom Alleviation

MR. STRASSER'S DENIAL

"Mr. Strasser is fifty-eight. He has an inoperable squamous cell carcinoma in the right lower lobe, with mediastinal metastases," Dr. Schuyt whispered. "He's had radiation therapy and the primary tumor has reduced, but on the X ray, cavities are visible that are possibly necrotic. There's little chance of improvement, but he's adamantly optimistic that he'll get better. I'll have to gradually make clear to him what his situation is."

It was weekly rounds on the pulmonology ward, and we were just outside Mr. Strasser's room, bunched around the trolley containing the patients' case notes—Dr. Glas and Dr. Schuyt, the two pulmonologists, a medical student, a nurse, and me. Some departments had "paper" rounds during which the case notes, lab results, and the nursing records were discussed before the doctors actually examined the patients. The pulmonology department usually had no "paper" rounds, and discussion took place in the corridor, just before they went in to see each patient.

"Well, let's go in and see him," Dr. Schuyt said, as he closed Mr. Strasser's file. We went into the room and gathered around Mr. Strasser's bed. He sat up, eyes wide and hopeful, mouth set in a tense smile.

"Doctor?"

"How are you feeling today?" Dr. Schuyt asked.

"Excellent, Doctor. How were the X rays?"

"I've just had a look at them, and it seems as if the tumor has become slightly smaller. . . . "

"Smaller," Mr. Strasser repeated.

"Yes, but you can't see it really clearly because of the effect of the radiation on the surrounding healthy tissue. . . . "

"Healthy tissue."

"Yes, now we've tried just about everything that's possible, and we're going to have to see how best to alleviate pain and shortness of breath."

"As long as it gets better, that's the important thing, isn't it, Doctor?"

Dr. Schuyt leaned against the wall. "Look," he said patiently, "you've had radiation therapy, the whole dose. We can't repeat that. I've explained that, haven't I? The tumor is a bit smaller, but it's not going to go away. What we've been trying to do is to reduce it slightly or at least keep it stable. You understand that, don't you?" Dr. Schuyt looked penetratingly at Mr. Strasser; Mr. Strasser looked back with an innocent expression and said nothing.

A few days later, Mr. Strasser was discharged from the hospital and went home. Home care had been arranged, and Dr. Schuyt was to keep a close eye on developments through his outpatient clinic.

A few weeks later, Mr. Strasser was readmitted to the hospital because of weakness in his right leg. A scan revealed extensive spinal metastases, and it was decided to treat these with radiation therapy. Mr. Strasser's optimism was not quelled by this evidence of physical decline. Indeed, a casual observer would have thought that he had been admitted to the hospital for some minor problem in his leg that would be cured in no time with a bit of physiotherapy.

He did, in fact, receive physiotherapy to try to keep him as mobile as possible. He waited enthusiastically for the physiotherapist every morning and exercised with dedication. I frequently saw him, lurching down the corridor, supported by the physiotherapist. During visiting hours, he discussed plans for the coming years with his wife. It seemed as though he was oblivious of the rampant tumor in his lung and the metastases proliferating throughout his body that, the doctors were convinced, would kill him before the end of the month. When we visited him during rounds, we found him sitting on his bed, waiting, in his neat, striped pajamas, with his legs stretched out in front of him.

"Look," he said, beaming. "I can move it a bit more," and with visible effort, he lifted his foot a few centimeters from the bed and wiggled his toes. "You see, it's improving. It's getting better." He fixed Dr. Schuyt with wide, hopeful eyes, a tense smile on his white lips.

"Yes," said Dr. Schuyt, hesitating. "Look, we're trying to get the metastases in your back under control with the radiation therapy, but we can't get rid of the tumor. I've told you that before, haven't I? All we can do is try to alleviate the effects of the tumor. We can't cure you; you realize that, don't you?"

"Yes, Doctor, I know." He looked up at the group assembled around his bed. "As long as it eventually gets better, that's the important thing, isn't it?"

During this period, Dr. Schuyt had a number of discussions with Mrs. Strasser. She was very sober about her husband's condition. She was quite aware that he was incurably and terminally ill, and although this was not easy for her, she accepted the situation. However, she did not want to force him to face the facts. Dr. Schuyt agreed with her, and they decided to wait and see what happened.

During the next week, Mr. Strasser's leg improved greatly, and at the end of the week, he was discharged again. Two weeks later, however, the weakness returned and he was admitted once more. Another scan revealed that the metastases were spreading rapidly. During this hospitalization he contracted pneumonia, and the doctors began to suspect that this would be his last admission. Gerrit Knol, just back from leave and now the junior doctor on the pulmonology ward, tried to sound him out. Mr. Strasser was very clear: as soon as he was better, he was going home. But the pneumonia persisted, despite high doses of antibiotics. Gerrit told me that the tumor was maintaining the pneumonia. Mr. Strasser was now getting morphine because of increasing pain caused by the metastases.

THE REVERSAL

Gerrit talked to Mrs. Strasser every day. She was still reluctant to make any attempt to persuade her husband to face the facts of his illness, but she began to notice a change in his attitude. He had told her that he was starting to doubt whether he would ever recover, and he started talking about death. He had never previously talked about his illness to his wife or his children. It was now, also for the first time, that he asked Gerrit to increase the morphine because the pain was becoming unbearable. He told Gerrit that he "didn't want to go on." He had lost a lot of weight; the contours of his skull had become visible, and his eyes were sunken in their sockets. He was agitated and kept picking invisible objects out of the air above his bed—something that was common among patients on high doses of morphine.

"How are you feeling now?" Gerrit asked him one morning.

"Okay, Doctor," he said.

"What are we going to do? Can you still manage?"

"We'll persevere," he said, with a tight, forced smile. "I'm getting penicillin, and as soon as the coughing stops, I'll be okay."

Gerrit visited Mr. Strasser every afternoon and tried to gauge whether there was any change in his attitude, as Mrs. Strasser had suggested, but each time he encountered only denial. Mrs. Strasser continued to claim that her husband's attitude was changing and that he had said that he did not want to go on, and the nurses now also started to tell Gerrit that their patient wanted to die. He had said that he was tired and didn't want to suffer any longer.

Then, a week later, Mrs. Strasser came to see Gerrit in his office. "Now he's *really* had enough," she said, "and he's been saying so for hours. He's asked to see the children and grandchildren so that he can say good-bye."

They then both went to see Mr. Strasser. "How are you feeling?" Gerrit asked.

"I can't take it anymore. I'm not going to get better. It's enough. I don't want to suffer like this anymore."

When Gerrit visited Mr. Strasser again later that evening, he got the same reaction. Gerrit then telephoned Dr. Schuyt, the specialist directly responsible for Mr. Strasser's treatment, and told him that there had been a reversal in Mr. Strasser's attitude, that he now wanted his suffering to end.

The next afternoon, Dr. Schuyt also went to talk to Mr. Strasser, who repeated that he had had enough and did not want to suffer any more pain. Dr. Schuyt said that he would increase the morphine. On June 15, 1992, Gerrit wrote the following:

Has requested that his life be terminated *[levensbeëindiging]*.[1] Request seems to be persistent. Has discussed this with wife and daughter. Said good-bye to family. Dr. Schuyt agrees. Start morphine, Valium, if necessary, in case of restlessness.

The next day, the report read as follows:

(4:00) Seems to come to occasionally. Unpleasant for the family (for us as well).
Morphine increased, after that tranquil.
(6:00) Passed away.

GERRIT KNOL'S INTERPRETATION

After the weekend, on June 20, I interviewed Gerrit Knol and asked him for his views on Mr. Strasser's death.

"I already knew that denial played an important role," Gerrit said, "particularly regarding the final stages. He never discussed his wishes or fears or feelings with his family. He simply repressed it, even though he had been told countless times what was happening. And . . . well, we let him go on denying: it's a well-known psychological mechanism.

"I tried to gently probe and find out what he really thought. He made it clear that he wanted to go home as soon as his condition permitted. That was initially what we were aiming at as well. But then, well . . . he was in such bad shape that his condition didn't improve, in spite of all the antibiotics. And he was already receiving high doses of morphine for the pain. That was because of the spinal metastases, for which he'd received the radiation therapy. He'd already had the optimal treatment for that, and, well, we knew he was going to die soon.

"We had discussions daily, and then we started to get the signal, through his wife, that he'd started to doubt whether he'd ever get better and whether he wanted to go on. I went to see him every afternoon to find out how he felt and whether he could still manage, without saying explicitly that he was terminally ill. But he kept insisting that he wanted to go on and that he was going to get better. So he kept denying.

"That happened two or three times, with the same result. But at the same time, his wife was bringing me a different message. Apparently, he didn't want to tell me that he thought he wouldn't be able to go home anymore. Then eventually his wife came to me to say that now he *really* didn't want to go on and that he had said good-bye to his children and grandchildren. So we went to see him, and it was now, for the first time, that he also told me that he couldn't cope anymore and that he'd had enough. So I called my boss, Mart Schuyt, and told him of the developments. He was aware of the whole history of denial, but now the reversal was very clear. Schuyt went to see him that afternoon, and he repeated what he had told me, and . . . well . . . we started with intravenous morphine, with the intention of letting him go to sleep [*inslapen*]. I discussed it with the family.

"I think it was realistic of him, and I could emphasize. He was bedridden, in pain, and had a serious pneumonia, as a result of which he was coughing up a lot of sputum, in spite of treatment. That was because of the tumor, which was keeping the pneumonia going. So I could understand that it was unpleasant, nasty for him. It was quite acceptable that he requested euthanasia [*levensbeëindiging*].

"It was also striking that he had been restless and hallucinating because of the morphine he was getting, but from the moment that the euthanasia arrangement had been made, he became tranquil. That wasn't only my impression, but also that of the nurses and his family.

"Then, unfortunately, we started with a morphine drip at a bad moment: Friday afternoon. But what else could we do? If there's a request like that, then we can hardly delay it until Monday morning because . . . because it's not convenient. You have to go through with it, I think. And although you have to burden your colleagues with it, it's part of the job, and most of us have had some experience with it.

"Mr. Strasser's condition gradually deteriorated, and the morphine was increased progressively. Eventually, Valium was added—I've mentioned that before, haven't I, that we sometimes use that combination?—and he passed away the next morning."

"What did you report as the cause of death?" I asked.

"A natural death," Gerrit answered.

"You mean that he died as a result of his illness?"

"Yes," Gerrit said. "I discussed the matter with Schuyt: whether we should inform the public prosecutor or get a second opinion, but he didn't think it was relevant. He saw it as a continuation of the treatment we'd already been giving him, which would have led to respiratory insufficiency anyway. Because that's the immediate cause of death: the morphine inhibits respiration to such an extent that it eventually stops altogether.

"But I did discuss the matter with him, I must admit, because you never make decisions like that alone. They [the specialists] have known the patients for much longer so we always discuss it with them."

"So the actual cause of death was respiratory insufficiency?"

"Yes, as a result of a metastasized lung carcinoma. That's what we fill in."

"Why do you think that Schuyt didn't consider it to be euthanasia? It could be interpreted that way."

"I don't know. Maybe you should ask him. . . . I think, and I've told you this before, that it's because it causes a lot of extra work and bother and nasty situations. You have to explain yourself to the public prosecutor. In the past, you could even expect police cars outside the door. You're more or less a suspect, and that's unpleasant for people who are just trying to do their job. And maybe the fact that it was Friday afternoon also played a role. Friday afternoons are difficult for decisions like that. But I think that Schuyt's main argument will be that it was simply the continuation of the treatment we'd already been giving, and I can understand that as well."

"Are junior doctors allowed to do things like that?" I asked.

"Yes, it's all part of our work. Schuyt gave me a lot of freedom to act as I thought fit. He said, 'Don't let it happen too quickly; otherwise, it'll look as though we really terminated him.' But that didn't happen. You want it to happen gradually—for the patient and for his family—because it can have emotional repercussions if the doctor just comes along, opens a tap, and the patient is dead in an hour. So we tried to let him go gradually."

"Did you give him anything else in addition to the morphine, like a muscle relaxant?"

"No, no, no, no. Well, Valium is a muscle relaxant. One of its effects is to relax the muscles. But we didn't give him one of the real muscle relaxants, like *Pavulon* [pancuronium bromide], no. But we don't use that. We use the benzodiazepines, the sedatives, that is, in large doses. Those and morphine, that's our most common combination."

"Why did you give him Valium? . . . That makes it look more like euthanasia."

"It depends on the situation. Maybe the patient isn't really short of breath, but he can have very superficial respiration and start *gasping,* as we call it. He can stop breathing for up to half a minute and then, suddenly, a gasp. It can last for ages, and just when the relatives think it's all over, he starts breathing again. It's not a pleasant sight. They can also turn blue, or fill up completely, because they can't cough up the mucus anymore. It differs from one patient to another. If the patient starts choking or panicking, then you have to do something."

"It seems to be a case that falls in the 'gray area.' "

"Yes, and if you report a case like that, then you're moving onto uncertain ground. They can be very mean if they notice that you haven't followed the rules to the letter. An action that one person interprets as *palliative abstention*[2] can be interpreted by another as euthanasia. The most important thing is that you try to act in accordance with your conscience. But that shouldn't be your only motivation. So, in that sense, I think that we need checks, but those checks are already there because you can never do something like that by yourself. There are the nurses, the specialists, other colleagues."

DR. SCHUYT'S INTERPRETATION

A week later I interviewed Dr. Schuyt. He was aware that I had spoken to Gerrit.

"I first saw Mr. Strasser . . . I think it was at the beginning of the year. He came to my outpatient clinic and there was an abnormality on the X ray. It soon became clear that he had a bronchus carcinoma. There was an enormous tumor load, a very big process in his right lung. The first option you look at is whether you can operate.

That wasn't possible. There was a very large tumor in the space between the lungs. The only thing we could do was radiation therapy, which helped slightly. But, as you could expect from such an extensive process, it was only temporary.

"The striking thing about Mr. Strasser was that he . . . well, he tended to repress it a little bit, in spite of that fact that I—and a lot of other people as well—kept telling him that the situation was bad. You heard him yourself, talking to his wife about plans for the next year, even the next five years, when that was totally unrealistic. And then there were the complications, which are quite common in cases like that: metastases in the spine, so neurological problems [sic]. Then only palliative measures remain. You have to make sure the patient isn't in pain. If necessary, you give radiation therapy, supplemented with pain medication, and you try to alleviate shortness of breath. In that stage there's no possibility of cure; you can only alleviate the symptoms, and that we did to the extent possible.

"But then what happens in cases like that is that you've just solved one problem when the next one appears. And the striking thing was that in spite of all this, he continued to deny that there was anything fundamentally wrong. It's a sort of defense mechanism, and I think that you have to give the patient enough room to digest the situation is his own way. There's no need to grab them and shake them and say, 'Now listen to me . . . ' So he repressed everything, right up to his final admission, even right up to the end of the final admission. . . ."

"What about his family?"

"They didn't repress it at all. I spoke to his wife on a number of occasions, and she realized, I think, that it was a hopeless situation. You can never say with certainty how long it will take because that can vary from one individual to another, but you can make it clear to them that it's a question of months rather than years.

"It was difficult for them that he repressed it like that and kept talking about next year. And that went on right up until the final admission, when you could really see him deteriorating daily. It was a completely metastasized lung cancer that required more and more morphine.

"Then, on Thursday, he stated clearly for the first time—to Gerrit Knol in the first instance—that he didn't want to go on anymore.

That was the moment that he seems to have more or less given up. So when you've tried all the palliative means at your disposal, and you see the patient deteriorating rapidly, and he repeatedly says that he doesn't want to go on, then you have to listen to him. His family had been ready for some time, but now he was also ready. I spoke to him on Friday. He was in really bad shape, and we agreed to give him morphine in a different way, a much larger dose, so that he wouldn't have to suffer anymore. So you increase the morphine with pain alleviation, dyspnea alleviation, in mind, and the patient doesn't suffer—at least we don't think he does. And so he passed away peacefully the next day, Saturday morning, I believe."

"Was the larger dose of morphine given with the *intention* of hastening death?" I asked.

"In that phase of the illness it was intended to . . . alleviate suffering. Because you could see that every movement, everything, was painful; you could see that he felt absolutely horrible. But when you do that you know that death will also be hastened: that's inevitable. But it's only a question of days, maybe a week or a week and a half at most, given the rapid progression of the disease. So you come to a decision that it's pointless to impose those few extra days of suffering. It's a common situation in lung cancer patients: increasing the pain and dyspnea alleviation in the knowledge that the patient will die sooner than he would have done if you didn't increase it."

"Did you give anything in addition to the morphine?"

"Only morphine, but then a larger dose and administered parenterally. And he was already getting large amounts orally."

"And you don't consider that to be euthanasia?"

"No, it wasn't euthanasia, no. I consider it to be. . . . It's something we frequently see in lung cancer patients: incurable, metastasized throughout the body, no chance of improvement, progressive deterioration, and increasing pain and dyspnea that you have to alleviate. And we do that radically, knowing that we are simultaneously hastening death, but having no choice. And that's not euthanasia."

"But imagine that the whole process had been exactly the same, but that he had gone on repressing right up until the end and hadn't said he was ready to die. Would you have acted in exactly the same way?"

"No . . . though, I must admit, he wouldn't have lasted very much longer anyway."

"But would you have given him as much morphine?"

"He was already getting a lot. But, in that case, we would have probably increased it more gradually. As it is, we did hasten the process, yes, consciously. But, in the last instance, it's the patient's wishes that are decisive."

"If you consciously speeded things up a bit, why wasn't it euthanasia?"

"Because it was primarily symptom alleviation. Look, if the dyspnea is so extreme then there's no other option, you could give him oxygen, but that wouldn't relieve the feeling of asphyxiation. Morphine is the only means of relieving that feeling, and that also hastens death. You've no alternative, and *that's* why I don't consider it to be euthanasia."

"So what would have to be different in order to have made it euthanasia?"

"There are a lot of patients in our practice with progressive lung emphysema, with a very poor lung function, and when that deteriorates further, their condition is at least as bad as Mr. Strasser's was. It can go on for a year, five years even. And if one of those patients says that he's had enough and doesn't want to go on, and you intervene, then *that* would be euthanasia. That's a different situation from Mr. Strasser, who was clearly in the very final stage of his illness. He only had a couple of weeks left at the very most, and in a case like that, your decision to intervene means that the patient dies tomorrow instead of next week. If you intervene in the case of the emphysema patient who would otherwise live for a few more years, then that would be euthanasia.

I haven't had many requests like that, although patients often hint in that direction, but cases like Mr. Strasser are very common on pulmonology wards. They're completely different situations, even though the degree of suffering is the same. But what can you do? There are hundreds of people with such limited lung function that all they can do is sit in front of the television all day; they're exhausted if they walk from their chair to their bed. They live like that for years, and many people think that they suffer unbearably as well, but you can't start giving them all large doses of morphine, can you?"

"Would it have been euthanasia if you'd given him a muscle relaxant, together with the morphine?" I asked, a bit provocatively.

Dr. Schuyt chuckled. "Yes, I think that, in that case, strictly speaking, you might be able to call it euthanasia. But you don't need euthanasia in situations like that because the patient is in the very final stage and is so weak that an increase in the morphine is enough. If you have a patient in physically better shape, then just increasing the morphine wouldn't be enough, and you'd have to give him something else as well, and that would really be euthanasia. That's no longer symptom alleviation with an earlier death as concomitant factor."

"But you could give Valium in addition to the morphine because he was restless . . . ?"

"Yes, yes, okay." Dr. Schuyt leaned back in his chair and laughed.

"In the case of euthanasia, you're supposed to get a second opinion. What do you do in cases like this? Do you also consult a colleague, or do you just make the decision yourself?"

"You discuss things with colleagues, with the ward doctor: you know the system here. It ensures that nothing funny happens. But, in the final instance, you make the decision yourself. It's essential, though, that you know what the patient himself wants, or would have wanted. The opinions of the relatives are important as well, of course, but that's not the most essential factor. I have a patient attending my outpatient clinic at the moment. She's not seriously ill yet, but she's already made her request for 'when the time comes'—I hope it never comes to that, but anyway—and we've arranged a meeting with a colleague, just to get things documented so that we're prepared if she's suddenly admitted and sticks to her request. In cases like that, you *have* to involve someone else. But that's really euthanasia. In the case of Mr. Strasser, I basically made the decision myself. It wasn't difficult; the situation was clear. There are much more difficult cases in which the line is not all that clear at all."

WAS IT EUTHANASIA
OR JUST SYMPTOM ALLEVIATION?

From the explanations of Gerrit Knol, the ward doctor, and Dr. Schuyt, the specialist, it is clear that Mr. Strasser's death was consciously hastened, although only by a few days. There are, however, striking differences between their interpretations. Gerrit interpreted the events leading to Mr. Strasser's death as euthanasia. Indeed, some of his statements give the impression that speeding up Mr. Strasser's death was the primary intention behind increasing the morphine. At one point, Gerrit described how Mr. Strasser was given morphine "with the intention of letting him go to sleep [*inslapen*]."

Gerrit's whole discourse suggests that he *expected* a request for euthanasia; it was just a question of *when* Mr. Strasser would give in and make it. The breakthrough came when Mrs. Strasser reported that her husband had started to doubt whether he wanted to go on. Gerrit went straight to Mr. Strasser to hear for himself, but Mr. Strasser maintained his denial. This apparently did not cause Gerrit to wonder whether Mrs. Strasser had, perhaps, interpreted the signs incorrectly, and he interpreted Mr. Strasser's reaction as fear of admitting that he was ready to die. Gerrit even went back regularly to see whether Mr. Strasser had changed his mind.

It would be going too far to claim that Gerrit was provoking a euthanasia request, but he was actively giving Mr. Strasser enough opportunity to express that wish, if he felt so inclined. He also had no difficulty in interpreting Mr. Strasser's request not to "suffer any longer" as a euthanasia request. "It was quite acceptable that he requested euthanasia [*levensbeëindiging*]," Gerrit had said, whereas Mr. Strasser had, as far as I was aware, never actually used the word euthanasia *(levensbeëindiging)*.

Gerrit saw this interpretation as being confirmed when Mr. Strasser summoned his children and grandchildren to say good-bye. (Formal leave-taking was a common way for terminally ill patients in this study to make clear that they were ready to die.) He saw further confirmation in the fact that Mr. Strasser appeared to become tranquil once they had promised to increase the morphine. (It was also not uncommon that patients who had struggled against their illness and resisted death almost until the end, suddenly gave up and then wanted to die as soon as possible. Once the doctor agreed to assist them, they became tranquil.)

When I asked Dr. Schuyt whether the increased morphine was consciously intended to hasten Mr. Strasser's death, Dr. Schuyt answered that it was primarily intended to alleviate his suffering, but with the knowledge that it would hasten death as well.

Dr. Schuyt placed a lot of emphasis, as did Gerrit, on what the patient, himself, wanted. Mr. Strasser said that he did not want to suffer anymore, and Gerrit interpreted that as a euthanasia request. Dr. Schuyt was more reserved in his interpretation, but both doctors' actions were motivated by the patient's wish not to suffer any longer, and with the same result: increased morphine, leading to an earlier death. They also both agreed that they would not have increased the morphine that much, or that quickly, if Mr. Strasser had not made his request.

At the end of my interview with Dr. Schuyt, I tried to explore the line between cases such as this and (what Dr. Schuyt would consider to be) euthanasia. From his remarks about patients with emphysema, it is clear that it is not only the wishes of the patient that are decisive in the decision to grant a euthanasia request but also the patient's life expectancy.

I tried to provoke Dr. Schuyt by seeing how far I could go in making hypothetical alterations to Mr. Strasser's situation before Dr. Schuyt would interpret his actions as euthanasia. If they had given him a muscle relaxant, then it would have been euthanasia, Dr. Schuyt said. Gerrit had given Mr. Strasser Valium, which is also a muscle relaxant. When I pointed this out, Dr. Schuyt only laughed, probably realizing in which direction I was leading him. Gerrit had already explained the reasons for giving Valium and the differences between that and the real muscle relaxants, such as Pavulon. Dr. Schuyt added that Mr. Strasser's condition was so bad that Valium would not have been necessary to hasten his death.

Although it is clear from Gerrit's discourse that he interpreted Mr. Strasser's death as euthanasia, he also did not seem to have any difficulty with the fact that Dr. Schuyt thought it unnecessary to report it as such. Part of his explanation is the general distaste for the "bother" that this would entail. Moreover, he was also sensitive to Dr. Schuyt's argument that it was not really euthanasia after all, but simply a continuation of the palliative treatment they had been giving. On the other hand, the very fact that he asked Dr. Schuyt whether they should report it confirms that he did think it had been euthanasia.

These different interpretations are also related to differences in personality and personal attitudes toward euthanasia. Dr. Schuyt considered euthanasia to be legitimate under certain conditions, and if those conditions were met, he was willing, in theory, to grant a request. He did so reluctantly, however. In fact, I had the impression that he actively tried to avoid it, if at all possible, without causing undue suffering to his patient. When, during the interview reported earlier, Dr. Schuyt mentioned a patient in his outpatient clinic who had requested euthanasia "when the time comes," he said that he hoped it would never get that far.

Gerrit, on the other hand, was almost eagerly awaiting a reversal in Mr. Strasser's attitude, and he tried to give Mr. Strasser enough opportunity to make a request, if he should feel so inclined. Dr. Schuyt would not ignore or "not hear" a legitimate request from a patient, nor would he take so much trouble to create suitable conditions for the expression of a potential request. For Dr. Schuyt, euthanasia was a necessary evil, something to be avoided, if at all possible; for Gerrit, it was part of his job, and if it enabled him to deliver a patient from suffering, then it was a satisfying part of his job.

Dr. Schuyt was right that they *could not* have acted otherwise. Mr. Strasser had clearly stated that he did not want to suffer any longer. Whether he really meant that he wanted to die or just wanted relief from suffering was irrelevant: the only possible relief the doctors had at their disposal would also hasten his death. Dr. Schuyt said, "Don't let it happen too quickly; otherwise, it'll look as though we really terminated him," but this does not mean that he really saw it as some sort of euthanasia, but simply that he started giving morphine in the knowledge that it would hasten Mr. Strasser's death, and he wanted to keep the extent of that hastening limited.

From a legal perspective, it is the doctor's *primary intention* that is decisive. It is clear that Dr. Schuyt's primary intention was the alleviation of suffering. If we assume that Gerrit's primary intention was the hastening of death, how should this be interpreted? As specialist in charge of Mr. Strasser's treatment, Dr. Schuyt was ultimately responsible for the decision, but Gerrit actually carried out the actions that hastened death. Moreover, if Dr. Schuyt's primary intention had been to hasten Mr. Strasser's death, but his actions had, at the same time, been the only ones that were medically acceptable (i.e., that it would have been medically and ethically unacceptable not to increase the morphine), would that have been euthanasia? And, would Dr. Schuyt have been liable to legal action?

Chapter 5

Coping with Pressure from the Family

MRS. LANSER

One morning, I was chatting to the secretary in the pulmonology outpatient clinic when Gerrit Knol, the ward doctor, came into the office and started rummaging through the files. After a few minutes, he found what he was looking for and prepared to leave. He paused in the doorway, the door half open, door handle in his hand, and said, as though he had only just noticed me, "Where the hell were you? I've been looking for you. There's been a lot happening on the ward. Mrs. Lanser has asked for euthanasia. The request came on Sunday, but the duty pulmonologist didn't want to make a decision, and I couldn't make a decision either. I've just been accosted by the nurses. They said, 'Something must be done urgently about Mrs. Lanser, and rather now than tomorrow.' I told them that I'm not the one to make the decisions and that they'd better wait for Dr. Glas."

After Gerrit had left, I went to the ward. In the doctor's office, I opened Mrs. Lanser's case notes:

> Sunday, 17 June, 10:30
> Has requested euthanasia. Has had enough.
> Not too short of breath.
> Husband supports her request. Children to visit.
> Terminal emphysema (and depression?).
> Discuss with pulmonologist.
> DNR [do not resuscitate]

The notes were written in Gerrit's hand. The file also contained letters—correspondence between Dr. Glas and Mrs. Lanser's GP. I paged through them.

Background: chronic respiratory insufficiency as a result of COPD [chronic obstructive pulmonary disease] (emphysema), for which she had been receiving oxygen. Whole series of admittances from 1983 onwards, mainly because of shortness of breath. . . .

From 9-10-90 to 24-12-90 admitted, initially in IC [intensive care], later pulmonology. Reason: the last few days progressive dyspnea . . . extremely dyspneic, cyanotic lady. She could hardly say more than a few words. Rehabilitation very difficult. Her complaints regarding shortness of breath also have an emotional component. She is uncertain about her own abilities, and this has led to her adopting the wrong breathing technique. . . .

From 2-3-91 to 30-3-91 again admitted to our unit. Once again, increased dyspnea, in spite of doxycycline and prednisone. The bronchial infection was treated with cefuroxime.
Once again, nervousness, lack of self-confidence, and family problems were important factors.
During this admission the patient spoke to the psychologist, and the physiotherapist gave her exercises. . . .

Mrs. Lanser was a small, fragile woman with a pale complexion and hollow cheeks. I initially estimated her to be in her late sixties, only to discover that she was fifty-five. She had aged prematurely as a result of the ravages of her disease. She had been admitted to the hospital in May because of shortness of breath and nervousness. Soon after, she contracted pneumonia, an illness from which she suffered frequently, and from that moment until her first explicit euthanasia request, she continued to become progressively more short of breath. This became so serious that she could no longer get out of bed to go to the toilet without assistance, and she was even out of breath if she turned over in bed. Dr. Glas told me that her lungs were so bad that "she hardly had any lung function left at all." I had seen her often during rounds, propped up with pillows, panting for breath, in spite of the oxygen she was receiving through nasal cannulas.

I was still paging through her file when Dr. Glas came into the office and asked me whether I was coming along to see Mrs. Lanser. She was awake when we entered her room, and Mr. Lanser was sitting next to the bed. Dr. Glas asked how she was feeling.

"I can't take this anymore," she said in a whisper. "I'm so tired of fighting, now I just want to die. . . . If the window was open and I could get out of bed, I'd jump." This she repeated several times during our visit.

"She's not sleeping anymore," Mr. Lanser said. "She hasn't slept for four days now."

"I understand your wish, and I support you completely," Dr. Glas said. "Your body is worn out, and we can't do anything more to help you. This suffering has become hopeless." Dr. Glas stood next to the bed, close to Mrs. Lanser. She clasped his hand with both her hands. Her fingers were long and white. Mr. Lanser stood on the other side of the bed, opposite Dr. Glas. He was crying. "I agree with her, Doctor," he sobbed. "I know it sounds terrible. I don't want to lose her, but this suffering must come to an end. I can't take this any longer either."

Dr. Glas repeated that he supported her and told her that he was going to do something. He said he would come back later to discuss things with the whole family. He told her that she need not be afraid, that she would not have to suffer much longer, and that dying was just like going to sleep. He gave a long and detailed explanation of the dying process.

When we returned, late in the afternoon, Mrs. Lanser's daughter and son-in-law were also there. While we were there, her son arrived. Mrs. Lanser was asleep, and it was the son-in-law who spoke for the family. He grilled Dr. Glas about Mrs. Lanser's chances of recovery. When Dr. Glas had explained why this was not an option, the son-in-law made it clear that the family had decided that if she was incurably ill, then there was no need to drag things out, to make her suffer unnecessarily. When the son-in-law had stated his case, everybody nodded solemnly, and a tense silence followed.

"There's no need to drag things out," Dr. Glas agreed. "I'll give instructions to stop all medication, except what is necessary for symptom alleviation, and I'll increase the oxygen. That will cause her to drop peacefully into a CO_2 narcosis."

At this announcement, everybody breathed a sigh of relief, and the atmosphere suddenly relaxed. The whole meeting had taken almost an hour.

"Is it going to take long?" the son-in-law asked as we were about to leave.

"I'm going to give instructions to stop unnecessary medication and increase the oxygen right now," Dr. Glas said. "I can't say exactly how long it will take before she passes away: it could be an hour, or it could take much longer, but I don't think it will be much longer than forty-eight hours." He moved toward the door, hesitated, and turned around. "I might as well alter the oxygen myself," he said. He walked over to the tap on the wall above Mrs. Lanser's bed and adjusted it. I heard another sigh of relief. I had the impression that they thought that Dr. Glas had made some magic gesture that would instantly deliver them from their misery. We then went back to the office, where Dr. Glas wrote the following in the file:

> Treatment options have been exhausted. Agree completely with her desire to stop treatment because this pointlessly delays her inevitable death, without diminishing the hopelessness of her situation or improving her quality of life at all. She is ready for death and longs for sleep. Consensus among patient, family, and doctor. Is expected to slip easily into an irreversible CO_2 narcosis.

Tuesday, June 19, 1991

When I came onto the ward the next morning, Gerrit said that the nurses had told him that the Lanser family was dissatisfied because the process was taking too long. "They'd expected it all to be over in an hour, but it's been twelve hours, and she's still alive," Gerrit said. "The family is exerting a lot of pressure. They want things speeded up. Mr. Lanser just said to me, 'You wouldn't let even a dog suffer like that; you'd put it to sleep.' I told him that I couldn't make any decisions."

I remarked that he seemed more reserved than in the case of Mr. Strasser.

"Yes, look," he said, "in the case of a terminal lung cancer like Mr. Strasser, the situation is clear. Someone like that is definitely going to die in the very short term. Situations like Mrs. Lanser's are

much more complicated. She's also suffering but could theoretically live for quite a while yet. And you can't be sure that you've *really*
done everything possible to pep her up, even if it's only temporary."

"She seems very nervous," I said.

"That's another thing we must take into account, I can tell you.
There's a psychiatric history there, and that was part of my problem,
on Sunday, when she suddenly said, 'Okay lads, I've had enough
now.' And then there's the husband, also exerting pressure, saying
things like, 'You wouldn't let even a dog suffer like that.' You have
to resist things like that. My answer was, 'I can't and I don't know.'
That's when I wrote 'Is she perhaps depressive?' in the file."

Later that day, I asked Connie, one of the nurses, whether the
Lansers were bitter because they thought that things were taking too
long. "No, not anymore," she answered. "I've had a talk with
Mr. Lanser to find out exactly what they want, and he said that as far
as he was concerned, things were okay, as long as his wife wasn't in
pain and as long as he didn't have the impression she was suffering.
This morning Glas also told them that things must take their natural
course. And, as it is, they are taking their natural course. I think that
as long as she remains in her present state, they're satisfied."

Wednesday, June 20

At half past eight in the morning, I was in Dr. Glas's office. He
told me that the nurses had phoned him the previous evening to say
that the Lanser family's mood kept changing: one moment family
members seemed to accept the situation, the next they were impatient. Dr. Glas told me that he would have to make clear to them that
things might go on for quite a while yet.

After leaving Dr. Glas, I went to the ward and opened Mrs. Lanser's file. I read:

> Becoming more drowsy. Consult Glas.
> 20 mg [milligrams] of morphine every three hours. To be in-
> creased in case of thirst/fear/dyspnea.
> NB [nota bene], in case of problems, even at night, consult
> Dr. Glas.

I went out into the corridor, where a group of nurses were having
a discussion. One said that Mrs. Lanser's son had been complaining

that things were taking too long. Another said that Dr. Glas had told the family that it could take forty-eight hours before Mrs. Lanser died, but that they had interpreted this literally: "They thought it was going to happen at one o' clock, as it were."

The nurses told me that during the previous night, under pressure from Mrs. Lanser's son, they had had a disagreement about what had been agreed. They phoned Dr. Glas at home. He was unable to come but informed the locum tenens, Rob Beenen, to give Mrs. Lanser 50 mg of morphine and possibly 20 mg of Valium. When Mr. Lanser realized that the locum tenens was going to increase the morphine, he intervened. *That* would be too much like euthanasia, he said. He said his wife did not seem to be in pain and that no increase was necessary. The locum tenens then decided to do nothing. The nurses now decided to reduce the previously agreed dose of morphine because they were afraid that she might die and that Mr. Lanser would accuse them of having euthanized her. They complained bitterly about Dr. Glas's instructions to increase the morphine "as and when necessary." How were they to decide? Why could Glas not simply state how much and how often?

They were still discussing this when Dr. Glas arrived on the ward. He said good morning, and the nurses returned his greeting. A silence fell. "Well, let's go and have a look," he said, and moved off in the direction of Mrs. Lanser's room. I followed. Mrs. Lanser was asleep. Around the bed, Mr. Lanser, their son, daughter, and son-in-law were gathered. They seemed calm but looked up expectantly at Dr. Glas. Dr. Glas explained that although it could be a while before she died, she was asleep and didn't seem to be suffering any discomfort. He dwelt at length on the dying process. The daughter was concerned about the possibility that emphysema was hereditary. Dr. Glas expanded on the nature and causes of the disease. Before leaving, he reduced the oxygen.

When we were outside, I said that I thought he was more reserved than in the case of Mrs. Van Nelle. I asked him what his reason was.

"The family," he said after a long silence. After another silence, he added, "Mrs. Van Nelle was a *very* different case. She was fully conscious, she was in pain, and suffering unbearably. With Mrs. Lanser it's different. She's asleep and doesn't feel a thing."

"Yes," I said, "but when we went to see her a couple of days ago, she was awake and suffering. She wanted euthanasia and even wanted to jump out of the window. Her husband agreed as well. I thought you'd take the same course of action as you did with Mrs. Van Nelle."

"There isn't a set of rules for cases like that; you have to judge each one separately."

Later the same morning, Gerrit came into the office. "What a mess last night," he said, as he dropped into a chair. "Glas apparently asked Rob Beenen to euthanize Mrs. Lanser. The husband intervened, and when I saw him this morning, Rob was furious with Glas." The phone rang, and Gerrit was called away to the emergency room. Shortly after, through the open door of the office, I saw Mr. Lanser running past. I got up and looked down the corridor in time to see Mr. Lanser and Janneke, one of the nurses, disappear into Mrs. Lanser's room. A while later, Janneke emerged and went to the medicine room. I followed and found her filling a syringe with morphine. I asked what was going on. She said that Mr. Lanser had panicked because his wife had opened her eyes. I asked her about the previous evening.

"They'd been complaining that it was taking too long," she said. "So we asked the locum to give her morphine through an infusion. He consulted Glas and then explained to the family that he wanted to start giving her morphine so that she could go to sleep. Mr. Lanser was opposed because it would be active euthanasia. Things have really been poorly arranged in this case. It was the same with Mrs. Van Nelle. But these aren't representative cases. Things usually go very smoothly."

Thursday, June 21

When I arrived on the ward the following morning, Gerrit informed me that Mrs. Lanser was dead. "Thank God," he added cynically.

Friday, June 22

In the evening, as I was about to leave, I passed Dr. Glas's office. I noticed that he was still in, so I went in and asked him what had happened on the evening that the locum tenens had attempted to increase Mrs. Lanser's morphine.

"The nurses called me," he said. "They said that the family was dissatisfied and they asked me whether things could be sped up. They'd been influenced by certain members of the family, you see, while other relatives had different views. So I phoned the locum and asked him to go and have a look. I said that, if he thought it necessary, he could set up an infusion and give her fifty milligrams of morphine, possibly supplemented with twenty milligrams of Valium. When he went to see her, he encountered a situation in which some of the relatives wanted him to act and others didn't. So, quite rightly, he didn't do anything."

I asked whose idea it had been to set up a morphine infusion, and he replied that it had been his.

Wednesday, June 27

The following Wednesday I had an interview with Rob Beenen, the locum tenens.

"I didn't know the patient at all," he said. "I didn't even know what was going on. Glas phoned me in the evening. He said it was a patient with terminal emphysema and that they had decided to abstain, that is, to stop all medication other that symptom alleviation. Glas had been phoned by the nurses, who had told him that Mr. Lanser was panicking and that things were going wrong. He told me that they were all waiting for her to die. She'd been receiving oxygen and morphine for a number of months. He said she was comatose and asked me to set up an infusion with morphine and Valium. I went to have a look, and the patient wasn't comatose at all. I woke her easily. The relatives got angry because I woke her up."

"Did you speak to her?" I asked.

"Yes, and she opened her eyes. She was very drowsy, but then the son-in-law pounced on me, so I didn't get a chance to ask her anything. I talked to Mr. Lanser, and he was in a bit of a state. He told me that they'd been expecting her to die for quite some time, but that she kept hanging on. The family had a discussion and couldn't agree on what should be done. Some of them thought that things should be slowed down. Mr. Lanser thought that they should be sped up. . . ."

"Who exactly thought that things should be slowed down?" I asked.

"The daughter. She was absolutely opposed to things being speeded up with an infusion. So I decided, seeing as I didn't know the patient, and also because I thought that it would have been a life-terminating act *[levensbeëindigend handelen]*, that I should refrain from doing anything, and that the attending physician—Glas—should sort things out. I explained the situation to Mr. Lanser, and he understood."

"So Mr. Lanser wanted things to be speeded up?"

"Yes, he insisted. He'd put pressure on Glas, through the nurses, to speed things up. But there was no consensus."

"Why were you dissatisfied?"

"I had the impression that it would have been a rather active termination of life. I could wake her easily, and she didn't seem to be terminal at that moment—in the sense of being on the point of death—and she didn't seem to be in pain or anything like that. I didn't know her, of course, but that was my first impression. So what could I do? I thought it was Glas's responsibility, and I thought that if I did it, it would be active euthanasia because she wanted to die. . . . I've experienced requests for euthanasia before, but they were handled differently. Colleagues were consulted, the public prosecutor was informed, a euthanasia declaration was signed: things that I didn't see recorded in Mrs. Lanser's file. I can imagine a person with terminal emphysema requesting euthanasia. Even when resting they feel like they're suffocating. I can imagine that they want to be relieved, but the proper procedure has to be followed."

MRS. JONAS

One morning, I was in Dr. Nieuwenhuis's endoscopy room. He had just finished examining a patient and sat with his back to me, writing his findings in the file. When he had finished, he closed the file and turned around.

"There's a woman on the ward who might become interesting for you," he said. "It's Mrs. Jonas. She's fifty-four. She underwent an operation for a colon carcinoma about five years ago. She's been suffering increasing pain in her right side for the last year. At the beginning of this month, she developed jaundice, and last week, she was admitted with various complications—probably liver metastases. There's not much we can do, and she'll probably not last very long."

Dr. Nieuwenhuis said that Frans Heine, the junior doctor, had spoken to her the previous evening, and he suggested that I go to see him.

"I told her that things looked bad," Frans said, when I interviewed him later that morning, "but that we'd only have the definitive results on Monday. She was in a lot of pain."

"How did she react?" I asked.

"It was really just a confirmation of what she already suspected. She wasn't surprised or shocked or anything. Of course, we'd already prepared her for the worst. You don't just do all those tests and then suddenly, out of the blue, tell her that it's serious. We knew from the scan and from other diagnostics that it could only be metastases, but the final proof can only come from cells under the microscope. She was already in the acceptance phase."

"Has she mentioned euthanasia?"

"No. Well, maybe indirectly, but certainly not explicitly. And she's the one who has to broach the subject. We can't push her in that direction. Sometimes she tells her husband that she doesn't want to go on, that she's tired and can't cope anymore. But she's afraid, I think, that we'll increase the morphine if she says that to us, and that she'll then have contributed to terminating her own life. That's the impression I have."

Monday, May 1, 1991

On Monday, the presence of metastases was confirmed, and that evening, Dr. Nieuwenhuis broke the news to Mrs. Jonas. He told her that the only course open to her now was palliation. Mrs. Jonas was calm and said that she had been prepared for the worst. "What I want to know now," she said, "is what's going to happen next. I want to know how things will end. . . . I *want* it to end as soon as possible."

"What do you mean?" Dr. Nieuwenhuis asked.

"I mean that I want to die as soon as possible . . . preferably a jab."

"Are you in a lot of pain?"

"No, not much pain . . . everything makes me tired, and this result has only increased that." She nodded toward her husband. "We've discussed things, and he agrees. I want to die decently. . . . I don't want to become emaciated. My sister died two years ago. She also had jaundice. She thought it was horrible. She said to me, '*Never* let this happen to you.' She'd had chemotherapy and was on painkillers that didn't help but only made her drowsy. They only drew out her suffering. . . . I don't want that to happen to me."

"If you want to end your life differently, then that can be discussed," Dr. Nieuwenhuis assured her. "But then you have to discuss it properly with everybody."

"I've already discussed it with my husband . . . but I don't want to talk about *that* with the children. . . . I *can't* talk to them about that. . . . I don't know whether it's possible . . . whether I'm allowed . . ." She fell silent. "I hope that God will just take me," she said after a while.

Later, when evaluating this discussion, Dr. Nieuwenhuis said to me, "She broached the topic of euthanasia but turned away from it again when she realized it could be discussed. She apparently found it too threatening. Probably because she thought that her children would be opposed. When I asked her, she just said, 'They won't be able to cope with it.' She didn't want her children to even *suspect* that she was contemplating it."

Mrs. Jonas could no longer eat and drink, and she now asked for the nasogastric feeding to be stopped. She also requested that all medication, except pain medication, be stopped. The pain medication was to be kept as low as possible because she did not want to be too drowsy either. It was agreed to increase the dose at night so that she could sleep. She was given a private room, and a second bed was installed so that her husband could join her.

It now seemed as though she had accepted things and was ready to die. "The struggle and the uncertainty have passed, even though her death sentence has been passed," one of the nurses said.

Saturday and Sunday, May 6 and 7

The more Mrs. Jonas accepted her situation, and the calmer she became, the more Mr. Jonas became impatient and emotional. This became acute on the weekend of May 6 and 7. Mrs. Jonas was experiencing increasing pain, for which she was receiving ever-increasing doses of morphine. She said that the situation was tolerable, but her husband began to complain that she was agitated and suffering unnecessarily. He repeatedly asked the nurses to increase the morphine even further. The nurses ignored these requests. To Frans Heine, the junior doctor, Mr. Jonas said, "She was so agitated last night. I think she's in pain. Can't you increase the morphine? She needn't know. We shouldn't burden her with the knowledge."

"Only your wife can make that decision," Frans had answered. "But she is drowsy because of the morphine, so we can't really ask her."

To me Frans said, "I think that he's more aware of how she's suffering than she is herself. But when he asks us to speed things up, we just have to ignore him. It's an issue in which he just has no say. You can't listen to the relatives in cases like this. You can only do what the patient, herself, wants."

"But he didn't explicitly ask you to hasten her death," I said.

"No, not really, but I think that that's what he meant. I think he's less religious than she is. I think that where there's life, there's still hope, even in situations like this. It's a difficult decision to make, to just throw the switch and say, 'Let me go.' Maybe she isn't ready yet. She knows that when she's taken that final step, she can't turn back."

Tuesday, May 9

On Tuesday, Dr. Nieuwenhuis informed me that Mrs. Jonas was feeling much better, even though she was still drowsy. "Contrary to her husband," he said. "He's putting increasing pressure on everybody to give her more morphine and hasten the end. It's not an uncommon phenomenon, to see a patient who is on the point of death suddenly recover and live for another few weeks."

"What exactly did Mr. Jonas say?" I asked.

"To me, not much. He's been talking to the nurses because he knows what my answer would be. I'd say to him, 'Sorry, your wife's the patient. She's breathing and you can communicate with her. It's unfortunate that she's in this condition, but you should be happy that she's still there at all.' I keep getting indirect signals from the nurses. It's difficult because they're also getting tired. . . . Then it's easy for a situation to develop in which the relatives and the nurses think that the doctors aren't doing enough for the patient."

"You mean hastening death?"

"Yes. They think you're letting the patient suffer unnecessarily. I can understand that, but it's the patient's choice. Perhaps everything has been muffled by the morphine and made tolerable. I think that she is quite capable of saying so, if she doesn't want to go on. But it remains difficult because she's in a sort of twilight situation. Yes, some people refer to increasing the morphine like that as passive euthanasia, but sometimes it's worse for the patient than when you do it actively. When the patient is fully conscious, you can say good-bye and really see them go to sleep. In the other case, the line is unclear, and the patient gradually slips away."

"Would she die that much sooner if you increased the morphine?"

"Difficult to say. I thought she'd have already died by now. She's not receiving any fluid because she's refused the infusion. In cases like that, you usually dehydrate fast. And then she's got a huge tumor, and pancreatitis, and jaundice. It's a mystery why someone in a situation like that *doesn't* die. I'm not sure whether the morphine would hasten things. Maybe things are taking longer *because* she's so calm. That happens as well."

Wednesday, May 10

When I arrived on the ward, a medical student informed me that there had been "problems" during the night. Mr. Jonas had complained that his wife was restless and demanded more morphine. The locum tenens had finally agreed.

Thursday, May 11

The following morning, I was met by the same medical student, who said that there had been "more problems" during the night. Mr. Jonas had demanded more morphine, together with codeine. He had said that his wife was restless and afraid. The nurses did not agree and had the impression that she was fast asleep and did not need anything. Indeed, Mrs. Jonas had refused codeine earlier because it made her too drowsy. The nurses had the impression that Mr. Jonas was a dominant man who was used to making decisions for his wife, and that he was now having a "mental breakdown."

Friday, May 12

Early Friday morning, Mrs. Jonas passed away peacefully in her sleep. Mr. Jonas and his children were reproachful. They thought that things had been allowed to drag on for too long. "They wanted everything to be sped up," Dr. Nieuwenhuis said, with a sigh, "but they didn't want euthanasia. People's expectations are often much too high. Sometimes they praise you, and sometimes they despise you," he said bitterly.

THE EUTHANASIA REQUESTS, THE RELATIVES, AND THE CONSERVATIVE OPTION

Mrs. Lanser's euthanasia request developed gradually after the last attack of pneumonia. During the course of several weeks, she repeatedly told the nurses that it was pointless to struggle on, since she would never get better. She seemed to gradually lose the will to continue. She said, "What difference does it make. If I improve now, it'll only be temporary. I'll be back in a month anyway, and what can I do in that month? When I'm at home, I can't even leave my bed. There's nothing that makes it worth hanging on." These remarks finally led to the urgent request to Dr. Glas on the eighteenth.

Mrs. Jonas also wanted to die but hoped that it would happen naturally. "I hope that God will just take me," she said. She frequently told her husband and the nurses that she had had enough and did not want to continue living, but when Dr. Nieuwenhuis informed her that she was free to request euthanasia, she closed the subject. It was clear, however, that she wanted to die; she refused all medication except that for pain alleviation, tube feeding and fluids in the full knowledge that this would hasten her death.

But she also wanted the pain medication to be kept to a minimum so as not to become drowsy. She knew that increasing the morphine would hasten her death, and Frans Heine interpreted her insistence that it be kept to a minimum as an indirect statement that she did not want to hasten her own death.

Both patients said that they wanted to die, but, for different reasons, their requests were not followed through. Shortly after she had expressed this request to Dr. Glas, Mrs. Lanser fell asleep and remained more or less on the sidelines until her death. Mrs. Jonas kept insisting that she wanted to die, but it was uncertain whether she really wanted active euthanasia. If she did, then she did not make this explicit enough for the doctors to be able to act.

When an individual becomes seriously ill, the social network which he or she is part of may be disrupted. If the pivotal member of the family becomes incapacitated, then the disruption is even greater, and mutual support may disintegrate. The opposite effect is also possible: that the members of a family or a social network move closer together, that the bonds between them become stronger, and that mutual support increases. In the first case, relatives argue and disagree about what to do, and friends keep away; in the second case, the relatives gather around the sickbed, and friends fly in from abroad. In the cases of Mrs. Lanser and Mrs. Jonas, both tendencies were present.

Mrs. Lanser's family drew together from the moment it became clear that she was terminally ill. The son, whom they had not seen for years, suddenly appeared and literally moved into his mother's hospital room, together with Mr. Lanser. They were there twenty-four hours a day, eating hospital food and taking turns sleeping on the spare bed in Mrs. Lanser's room. The daughter and son-in-law were also in the hospital most of the time that they were not working or taking care of their children.

When Mrs. Lanser made her euthanasia request to Dr. Glas, she was fully conscious and lucid, and everyone seemed to agree with her. Mrs. Lanser had always been dominant, and her husband and children had depended on her. However, when, shortly after making her request, she fell into a deep sleep, the one stable factor and the source of the euthanasia request disappeared from the scene. She became the "object" of a discussion about how long "it" should go on, and the opposing views of the various relatives began to emerge.

The son thought that things were taking much too long, and he repeatedly put pressure on the nurses to shorten his mother's life by increasing the morphine. And when the son-in-law spoke for the family, he also argued for hastening Mrs. Lanser's death. However, when the locum tenens came to install the morphine infusion, the daughter intervened because it would be "active euthanasia." Mr. Lanser fluctuated between these two extremes, depending on his mood and his wife's condition. When she was fully conscious and requested euthanasia, he agreed with her, and, later, when she seemed restless or opened her eyes, he panicked and demanded more morphine, but when he thought that she was calm, he did not think it necessary.

In the Jonas family, the social dynamics were somewhat different. Mrs. Jonas's two children came to visit her every day, but their sojourns in the hospital were limited to visiting hours. Although they did not seem to be any less caring than the Lanser children, there was a measured commitment of time rather than the unlimited commitment that characterized the Lanser children's response. This was partly because of the obligations of work and their own children, but also partly due to the fact that Mr. Jonas insisted on taking care of everything himself. He was always in the hospital, sleeping in his wife's room and attempting to maintain as much control over the situation as he could. He also wanted to keep his wife's desire to die hidden from their children, both of whom were very religious. I also had the impression that he was trying to hide from them the fact that he was putting pressure on the medical staff to hasten his wife's death.

Mrs. Jonas's euthanasia request was also different from that of Mrs. Lanser. Mrs. Lanser's request was clear and consistent, as long as she was physically capable of expressing it. Mrs. Jonas's request fluctuated. She wanted to die but was not sure whether she could justify euthanasia to her children or square it with her own religious conscience. Mr. Jonas was opposed to active euthanasia, but in spite of this, he wanted the doctors to hasten his wife's death. This was partly because he thought that she was suffering unnecessarily and partly because he could not cope emotionally with the drawn-out process of her dying. Their children were strict Catholics, so any discussion of euthanasia or hastening death was out of the question, and as Mrs. Jonas became increasing calm and resigned, Mr. Jonas increasingly had to cope with the problem by himself. This increased the emotional burden on him, and he seemed to become increasingly labile. In the later stages, he would run to the nurses in panic, demanding morphine, just because his wife had moved or made a sound in her sleep.

Both cases involved pressure from the relatives to speed things up, in the absence of a clear request (or confirmation of a request) from the patients: in the case of Mrs. Lanser, because she was asleep, and in the case of Mrs. Jonas, because she was inconsistent. Divisions and disagreements were also present among the relatives: some of Mrs. Lanser's relatives were opposed to euthanasia; Mr. Jonas was equivocal, and the children were opposed to euthanasia. The attitudes and wishes of individual relatives and social relationships between them, therefore, had an influence on the actions of the doctors, though this was not necessarily the effect intended. Far from leading to a hastening of death, pressure from relatives to speed things up led the doctors to become more conservative to draw back from actions that might be construed as euthanasia.

In the case of Mrs. Jonas, her unwillingness to explicitly request euthanasia when Dr. Nieuwenhuis confronted her, together with pressure exerted by Mr. Jonas and knowledge of their children's opposition, led to consensus among the care providers that no action should be taken. This occurred even though the care providers were convinced that Mrs. Jonas wanted to die and that she had proved this by refusing all treatment as well as nasogastric feeding and fluids. In the case of Mrs. Lanser, disagreements among the relatives in the absence of a clear input by the patient led to disagreements among the different care providers. This lack of consensus also led to no action being taken.

Chapter 6

A Reflexive Intermezzo

DIALOGUE

My approach in carrying out this study was both performative and dialogical. A dialogical approach implies that the "work of interpretation" is never complete (Tedlock 1983; Pool 1994). Dialogue with participants and with the texts of what they have said can be continued into the writing phase by letting the participants read what you have written about them and your interpretations of what they have said, letting them comment, and integrating those comments as well. The end product need not be a complete and polished picture but can allow some of the different and competing voices to be heard.

I had already tried this approach in a book on interpretations of illness and misfortune in a village in Cameroon (Pool 1994), but the feedback had been disappointing, in a largely illiterate setting, and the dialogue dried up once I left the field. However, when the plan for this book began to materialize during my research in the hospital, I decided to continue my Cameroon experiment in Randstad. I would make my interpretations and draw my conclusions, feed them back to the participants, and integrate their comments, interpretations, and criticisms into the text as part of a dialogical project.

After writing the first five chapters, I made copies and distributed them to the participants.[1] Here, I limited myself to the hospital staff and did not involve the patients and their relatives. The main reason for this selection was that the patients I had written about had all died recently, and I did not want to intrude on the friends and relatives yet. I was planning to discuss the whole manuscript with *all* participants once it had been completed. This never materialized, however, due to my moving on to another job in Tanzania before the manuscript was completed.

Another reason for handing out the first five chapters to the medical staff at this stage was, basically, uncertainty. I was worried that they would find what I had to say—and the way I said it—unacceptable, and that it would be pointless to write a whole book only to have it vetoed. Obviously, I was not prepared to tolerate censorship, but, from the start, I had decided that I would not go ahead and publish anything if there was fundamental resistance from any of the participants: medical staff, hospital administration, patients, or relatives. This decision was strengthened during the research when I saw to what extent participants took me into their confidence and shared their most intimate moments and thoughts with me, for the benefit of my study. On the other hand, I was also determined to write everything and present everything as I experienced it, warts and all. I was prepared to do my best to persuade everyone that that was necessary, but I was worried about anonymity. After five chapters, I needed a green light before continuing.

I had originally planned to be present during the discussions and to record them, but I had already left for Tanzania, and so a group of participants discussed the chapters without me. However, on their own initiative, they recorded their discussion and sent me the tape. The issues raised are important enough to justify inserting their discussion here, as transcribed from the tape, as an interim meta comment.

THE DOCTORS' DISCUSSION

Participants. Marthe Diepen (psychologist), Peter Glas (pulmonologist), Martin Schuyt (pulmonologist), Emiel Roelofs (internist), and Mieke Van der Ven (anesthetist) were present. Jan Smit (head nurse) could not attend but made written comments.

Marthe Diepen: I suggest we try and answer the questions as listed in his letter: He wants to know whether it's sufficiently anonymous. Do we agree with the way it's turned out on paper, given his premise that everything should be transcribed as literally as possible from the tapes? In summary, can we accept this form of presentation? And can we comment on the contents?

Martin Schuyt: It's recognizable, and I wonder to what extent the relatives are going to recognize things. It's all there, literally, exactly what happened. He's only changed the names, but the situations are exactly the same. That's different to what he did previously, in an experimental article in which he fictionalized the case studies —as he called it [Pool, 1992]. He conflated two patients and changed the medical specializations.

Marthe Diepen: Do you object to the way he's done it this time?

Martin Schuyt: I wonder whether the relatives will object. Of course, there was informed consent, but did they *really* understand? What about all the brothers and sisters and so on? Did they all realize that sooner or later it would all be in a book, lying there in the shop? I can imagine someone taking up the book and reading it and thinking, "Hey, that's me." He discussed it with all those directly involved, but the more distant relatives might have been lost sight of. So I wonder whether it will cause problems for the relatives.

Emiel Roelofs: Yes, I can imagine that when people read about how they're talked about. . . . For example, he writes somewhere that when a relative asked whether the doctor could give the patient a jab, the doctor says, "When she asked me that I thought, "Now I'm not going to do it." That could be nasty if the relative—

Martin Schuyt: Exactly.

Emiel Roelofs: . . . whose father or mother it was, read it.

Peter Glas: That's the disadvantage of presenting it literally. It would be better to see the quotations as the small type in a description of events. And they need situating. He should describe things rather than just let the events come at you like that. It all runs a bit too smoothly—

Emiel Roelofs: I don't agree. I think—and that's how he planned it—that he used himself as research instrument. It was *participant observation.* And I have to admit, he represents things uncomfortably accurately, at least, speaking for myself. I recognize myself immediately, not only the words I spoke, but his interpretation of my actions as well. It corresponds precisely.

Peter Glas: But that can be interpreted in different ways, and that's dysfunctional. The bit about his brief contact with Van Ham, for example. I'm not sure whether you can just put it in a book like that. It's illustrative of how some people communicate about these issues in certain situations, but if you want to present it, you have to annotate it with explanations—

Marthe Diepen: I don't think I agree with you. Listen, why did he do this research, and why is he writing this book? Precisely because it's an emotional subject and those patients know that we react emotionally to it, and that's a good thing. I *do* think that you must take into account whether you're saying things that would unnecessarily hurt someone's feelings, like some of his descriptions of individuals or relationships, which are summaries and interpretations after all. I have my doubts about that. But I don't mind patients reading about doctors reacting like Van Ham. We're human beings, after all. . . .

Peter Glas: Then it should be annotated as such. Well, I suppose he does do that in the second part of each chapter. But when you just read it like that, then it's open to multiple interpretations, and third parties can get the wrong impression. Jan said the same thing in his written comments. Of course, Robert saw it like that, and maybe he *has to* describe it like that, but if the relatives—

Marthe Diepen: What I find difficult is that we get a chance to comment on what he's written about us, but the patients and their relatives don't. Listen, there are things in there that I've said about some of you, for example, without you knowing what I thought. I told Robert those things in what I assumed to be a sort of relationship of trust, and then suddenly it's in print, and you read it and think, "Oh, I see. Is that what Marthe Diepen said about me?" [Everyone laughs.] Well, I can live with that, if it's something that I would have said to the person's face as well, except then I would have used different—

Peter Glas: He describes it from the perspective of ego. If the descriptions were more passive, then you could describe things like that, but they wouldn't be put directly in your mouth. Then nobody needs to feel that a finger is being pointed at them.

Emiel Roelofs: But I think that if the question is, "Is it acceptable like this?" Then the answer is, "Yes." But it has to be made more anonymous. He could make terminal emphysema into a terminal heart problem, for example. And he can change men into women.

Martin Schuyt: Fictionalization . . . yes. Because as it is, it's too precise. You should shuffle it about a bit. But that's tricky because you have to preserve the essence of—

Emiel Roelofs: But if he consistently falsifies the specializations: all pulmonologists become cardiologists, and all lung complaints become heart complaints—

Peter Glas: But that would be tricky. I've taught him quite a bit of the technicalities of my trade, and the rest of you have done the same, and it's difficult to alter the specifics of the various syndromes . . .

Marthe Diepen: But I know, for example, that morphine is used in one hundred percent of cases with terminal heart . . .

Mieke Van der Ven: You can only alter that professionally. Robert couldn't do that—

Marthe Diepen: Yes, because it has to be internally consistent—

Martin Schuyt: That's a problem.

Peter Glas: We could make suggestions.

Emiel Roelofs: Yes, everybody could take his own bit and tell him what can be altered and how because we have the knowledge.

Mieke Van der Ven: But aren't you then intervening too radically in his story, because now it runs so smoothly. You read through it just like that. But if you start altering things like that, then you get an adaptation, and I'm not sure that it won't turn out differently. He'd have to rewrite everything.

Marthe Diepen: Maybe we could make a selection and only change some things, or consult the relatives in cases we're not sure of? After all, they know that the study was carried out; they know a book is being written. We could say, "This is what's been written, and we're worried it might be unpleasant for you, so would you mind reading it?" We wouldn't have to do it for everyone—

Emiel Roelofs: But then the damage would already be done because they'd have read it anyway.

Marthe Diepen: But that's how things are.

Emiel Roelofs: That's why I think it's acceptable as it is, as long as it's made more anonymous. Changing the illness doesn't alter the essence, but it would make it less recognizable for the relatives—

Martin Schuyt: And change the times and dates: March becomes September, for example. Those aren't essential. . . .

Peter Glas: Yes, because you can't alter essential details.

Marthe Diepen: Some of the details that aren't essential could also be left out because they could also be experienced as unpleasant. It's like the right of inspection: you have a right to read your own case notes, *except* the personal notes. And what we're talking about here are personal notes. Why don't we let people read the personal notes? Because they're no use to them and might cause misunderstandings, and because they're not meant to be read by them. But, on the other hand, I think it's very clever, and I think we have to accept that he's writing it all down.

Peter Glas: We do, we do. I certainly agree with him.

Emiel Roelofs: Yes, we all agree on that.

Peter Glas: Then we must attempt to make adjustments here and there. I think that would help him.

Marthe Diepen: I also think he shouldn't use existing names.

Peter Glas: He can make it even more anonymous by just using initials. That's how we do it in the medical literature.

Marthe Diepen: Mrs. A., Mr. B. Alphabetic. [Noises of agreement]

Emiel Roelofs: And the sections that have been taken literally from the files, the case notes, and the nursing reports—I wonder whether that could be traced, in case of legal action. Some nitpicker could come along and spend a month going through the files. . . . But, on the other hand, those quotations *are* an important part of the story. He didn't select them for nothing. But they do make it more recognizable.

Peter Glas: It could be done more descriptively. He could write something like, "From the nursing report, it became apparent that the nurses were irritated by the fact that the doctor still hadn't been to see the patient." It could be stated more passively.

Marthe Diepen: But that would make it boring, which is what he's trying to avoid. And we did give him access to those files, and he is an anthropologist—

Mieke Van der Ven: It's his direct approach that's so gripping.

Peter Glas: Yes, but it could be qualified by an explanation.

Emiel Roelofs: Yes, but that would reduce the effect. As it stands, you can *feel* the irritation because Dr. So-and-So *still* hasn't come. And it happens, and it's important that it's said. . . . I'm just worried about some nitpicker—

Peter Glas: We have to take precautions.

Marthe Diepen: Yes, it's a small world, and there are people who know the study was carried out in this hospital.

Mieke Van der Ven: You might be reproached by colleagues: How can you say things like that as an anesthetist? You could say that you stood by the things you said, but. . . . Once I had a two-hour discussion with Robert—two hours of words, which he summarizes very well, but it hits hard. When I'm confronted with the things I said like that, I sometimes have to swallow hard. It makes you realize you have a lot to answer for, not only to yourself, but to colleagues as well. So I think it should be as anonymous as possible, without affecting the gripping story he has to tell because it *is* gripping. I managed to trace each and every situation. I kept thinking, "Oh, that's so-and-so, and this must be so-and-so." You tend to forget things as well, and in another couple of years, it will be even further away, but it's still a bit frightening.

Marthe Diepen: I had the same experience. Sometimes I thought, "Did I *really* say that?" When you see it in print like that it seems different. I thought, "When you transcribe things verbatim like that, to what extent do you represent what *really* happened?" I don't have an answer, but some things are much harder when they're in print than when you say them in a conversation.

Martin Schuyt: Sometimes we told him things while walking, running, from one ward to another, from one patient to another, and then suddenly you're confronted by those statements, hard as nails, on paper.

Mieke Van der Ven: That's what makes it so powerful. [Sounds of agreement]

Emiel Roelofs: Yes, because even if it was said while running and in a hurry, it wasn't said for nothing.

Martin Schuyt: Yes, that's true, yes.

Marthe Diepen: And the fact that, running and in a hurry, emotions are exchanged is also important.

Emiel Roelofs: I have to go, but I just want to say that I think it's acceptable like this, but it needs to be more anonymous. I don't have any problem with the verbatim reporting, as long as we're sure we won't be prosecuted.

Marthe Diepen: The director supports Robert completely, and before anyone can do any harm, he'd have to get support from the public prosecutor by convincing him that a punishable offense had been committed.

Emiel Roelofs: But someone who knows that the study was done in this hospital could report that we carried out euthanasia. . . .

Marthe Diepen: Maybe some of the cases have just been dismissed by the public prosecutor, and then the book gets published and he reads it and thinks, "Interesting. I recognize that case, but I wasn't aware of those details"—

Emiel Roelofs: The morphine was increased in some cases in which a natural cause of death was reported, and, well, that could be interpreted in various ways.

Marthe Diepen: That's well known.

Emiel Roelofs: We have to find out whether the cases described here are liable to prosecution.

Marthe Diepen: Can we find that out? We can ask Robert whether he has any ideas, and whether he can get advice from an expert. Do you also think we need legal support?

Mieke Van der Ven: Yes, and I think we have to ask the director explicitly what his position is.

Marthe Diepen: We need to know whether we can rely on the director's support as long as there's the possibility that someone can score by investigating things further.

[A long discussion followed about when it would be possible for each of them to send me their suggestions for increasing anonymity.]

Peter Glas: What I missed in the first chapter was a discussion of his research goals: what he wanted to find out. All he does is describe he actually did it.

Marthe Diepen: But that *was* his goal. He described his methodology, and the rest developed from there. That *was* the methodology, and he explains it. He describes his approach, but not what he would find, because that all depended on how things went. . . . If he's presented it chronologically, then what strikes me is that all the cases in which I was involved are at the beginning. I had the impression that the more he established a place for himself and became a confidant—

Martin Schuyt: The more he took over your role [laughs].

Marthe Diepen: . . . the less I was consulted. Precisely.

Peter Glas: Yes, that's quite likely.

Marthe Diepen: When you read in the file, "Dr. Pool to talk to the patient." Or whatever it was—

Peter Glas: Yes, but that was only on the odd occasion though. But on the other hand, we did make use of him as well.

Marthe Diepen: He did acquire a place in the whole—

Martin Schuyt: I think that there were certainly situations in which you would normally have been consulted, but that he was asked to talk to the patient instead.

Marthe Diepen: Yes, and with that in mind, he could say something more about our need to discuss such matters. I mean, the fact that he acquired such a role is not coincidental. And the fact that the doctors feel that need more than the nurses is also worth considering. We need to consider whether we interact adequately with each other in these matters. Is there a possibility, when you lie awake thinking of such matters, to talk to someone about it? Or, in the case of euthanasia or other difficult end-of-life situations, to sit down together for half an hour and discuss [it]. I've had that feeling, that I was glad that I ran into someone on the stairs, and then you just stand there and talk—

Peter Glas: Some of us do create situations like that. I see that among the nurses, that they feel the need and that we fail in our duty toward them.

Marthe Diepen: It illustrates the way in which doctors and nurses work alongside each other but not together, don't you think?

Peter Glas: Yes, you're right.

Marthe Diepen: And Robert needs to consider why it is that Jan thinks that the nurses' role in the book is too small. That also tells us something about the whole—

Peter Glas: We've discussed this before: who is most involved with the patient in crisis situations like that? Of course, you *do* communicate with the nurses about these matters, but only with those who are directly involved at that moment. And then suddenly, from a completely unexpected corner, others criticize your actions. You say, "We've discussed it," and you wonder whether they've communicated. Sometimes the communication isn't as good as it should be. And you also act defensively. It's easier to talk to a colleague or a junior doctor than to venture into the nurses' coffee lounge. That's something you only do sporadically.

Mieke Van der Ven: The funny thing is that because of his presence the discussions—

Peter Glas: Were *very* direct. Yes.

Mieke Van der Ven: I noticed that clearly in intensive care. On a number of occasions, there have been discussions resulting from things that happened, among the nurses, but also between the doctors and nurses. Extensive discussions. There were also discussions later, after he left, but they all referred back to that period. I think that an evaluation afterwards is important for everybody, for how you cope with what's happened, but normally there's nothing. There are always situations in which one person says this and another that and yet another something else, and that's what you read here in these pages. So it's good to discuss things more. Of course, it's not necessary that everybody agrees all the time, but too much disagreement can lead to misunderstandings.

Peter Glas: Yes, that comes out clearly in his performative approach, but because different interpretations are possible, it would be better if they were annotated so that you don't get wrong interpretations.

Marthe Diepen: I think that, whatever happens, his book is going to cause a lot of waves, and if someone has the wrong intentions, then you can't avoid that, however honest, however careful, however balanced you make it. And so I think we shouldn't be too hesitant. If we agree that it contains important information, inside information, which will be useful to others, if they make proper use of it, then we must be prepared to put up with the rest as well. It will be translated into American [sic], without a doubt, and it'll be used over there to show how terrible the situation is here [everyone laughs], but that's something we can't avoid. People who say, "It's unacceptable," will buy it and say, "You see, it's unacceptable," and people who want to learn something more about that sort of thing will buy it for that reason.

Martin Schuyt: It's difficult for us to estimate how people without any medical knowledge whatsoever, except what they've gleaned from *Emergency Room* [a Dutch daytime soap opera], will interpret it. Because it's written in such a way that you can do almost anything with it. You can find support in it for whatever you want to argue.

Peter Glas: Sometimes it is a bit like *Emergency Room,* isn't it?

Martin Schuyt: Yes, it definitely has a bit of everything, and we know in what sort of context to place it, but if you don't know anything about it, then that could lead to the wrong interpretation.

Marthe Diepen: Do you think there's too much description of cases?

Mieke Van der Ven: I did initially.

Marthe Diepen: That you reach saturation point?

Marthe Diepen: It is a concentrated dose of misery, isn't it? [Everyone laughs.] In *Emergency Room,* you also get a whole year's misery dished up in half an hour.

Mieke Van der Ven: What strikes me is that the last year has been so quiet as far as euthanasia goes. When I think about the last case of euthanasia I was involved in, I really have to think back. Whereas when Robert was here, I had the feeling that they were coming at me from every corner. If I ran into him and he asked me whether anything had happened, I would say, "You've missed this and you've missed that, but perhaps you can still catch this."

Peter Glas: Yes, you're right. That's how it was.

Marthe Diepen: But don't you think that it was his presence that made you realize how often it really occurred? Because there are a lot of situations which never end up as euthanasia, but he was interested in euthanasia cases and inquired about them, and so focused our attention on them. Sometimes he asked me whether anything had happened, and I was convinced that I hadn't forgotten to inform him, but then he would say, "What about so-and-so?" And then I thought, "Damn it, you're right." So it seems like I forget things like that relatively easily and have to be reminded.

Mieke Van der Ven: Yes, now that you mention it, when I think back over the last few months, I can recall three cases.

Marthe Diepen: I think we try to repress it.

THEMES

What follows is not meant to give answers to the questions raised by the doctors in their discussion (although I do provide some answers), but to point to some of the important themes that emerged.

The first thing that struck me, particularly in the first half of the discussion, was the anxiety about the possibility that the hospital or the participants might be recognized. This anxiety related to the threat of legal sanctions against the doctors and the possibility of emotional consequences for the relatives. Although the possibility of legal sanctions relating to some of the cases could not be excluded entirely, it was not very likely either, given the ambiguity of the situations in question and the gradually shifting line in Dutch jurisprudence between the acceptable and the unacceptable. However, only a few years had passed since doctors who carried out euthanasia could expect policemen in the waiting room, and not all doctors in the hospital were fully aware that this no longer occurred.

I had always explained what the study was about and asked permission before involving a patient in the study. In practice, it was also necessary to have the support of all the relatives who were directly involved as well. From the start, I had intended to include only those patients whose relatives supported participation unanimously. If one member of the patient's family was opposed, then the patient was excluded (this happened only once, however). Problematic issues relating to the exact nature of informed consent, still remain, however, as Dr. Schuyt points out in the discussion. In spite of all my explanations, to what extent did the relatives—and the patient for that matter—understand what was *really* going on, or what I was planning to do with my findings? I was not entirely sure what I was going to do with them myself. It was, after all, an exploratory study, and I was not sure what I was going to find.

It could be argued that it is unnecessary, from an ethical viewpoint, and impossible from a practical viewpoint, to have full informed consent in social scientific research, but there is consensus that some degree of consent is necessary. But where should the line be drawn? I had been prepared to go as far as possible in this. My plan was to use dialogue as a central concept and involve all participants in the study: patients, relatives, doctors, nurses, and so forth. I wanted them to read my descriptions and interpretations and comment on them so that I could include their voices, their interpretations, and their criticisms together with my own. The problems with this setup were practical. Whereas the care providers were always conveniently available in the hospital (even though this by no means meant it was easy to see them), this was not the case for the patients and their relatives. The patients with whom I had most contact and who were the central players all died before anything had actually been written about them, and my relationship with many of the relatives, although somewhat close during the period of crisis, disintegrated rapidly after the patient had died and their contact with the hospital was severed. The original plan had been to visit the families of the most important patients a year after the fieldwork had been completed, evaluate what had happened, and discuss my interpretations with them. This became impossible once I had left the country.

In their discussion, the doctors expressed much concern about wrong interpretations of their statements and the necessity of annotating what was said to provide sufficient context to avoid such misinterpretations. Their problem—that statements were open to multiple interpretations—was my epistemological point of departure. However much you contextualize and annotate, statements will still be susceptible to different interpretations. Stimulated by discussions in philosophy and literary theory, anthropological discussions have focused closely, during the past fifteen years, on representation. The extent to which descriptions (can) accurately represent social reality was questioned, and the traditional naturalistic and realistic genre conventions, adopted from premodernist literature and the biological monograph, were criticized. This led to a plethora of "experimental ethnographies" in which anthropologists experimented with various genres and styles of presentation. One of these was dialogue. Instead of describing what respondents said and interpreting it, their statements and interpretations are presented literally and can be compared directly to the author's interpretation. My own approach in this study was influenced by this dialogical anthropology.

In connection with dialogical anthropology, much discussion has focused on whether a text in the form of a dialogue is an accurate representation of the original dialogue, whether it provides an accurate representation of the culture and the ideas of the people studied, and whether such a text can be considered to be a real dialogue, given that the anthropologist has ultimate editorial authority (Clifford 1983; Tyler 1987).

One of the fundamental problems with much experimental ethnography, and with the whole discussion about the representation of culture, is the implicit assumption that the accurate representation of culture is the *goal* of ethnography.[2] My use of dialogues here is not meant to represent the actual dialogues in the hospital. That is impossible, if only because they have been recorded, transcribed, translated into English, selected, and edited. Other sounds, facial expressions, intonation, and gestures have all been reduced to a few descriptive phrases. Much of the context is gone, and only the words remain, and they have to carry the full load of meaning. The dialogues are meant to evoke situations in the hospital: how people talked about euthanasia, what they did, how they coped. They are also meant to evoke *my experience* of that.

Despite believing that statements are always open to alternative interpretations, I assumed that recorded statements transcribed verbatim were more "accurate" than what was merely remembered by the participants. At one point, Marthe Diepen says that "some things are much harder when they're in print than when you say them in a conversation." Sometimes, when I reread the transcripts of conversations, I had a similar experience: the literally transcribed statements seemed different from what I remembered. What should we do with such statements? Should they simply be presented verbatim, or should we alter them to bring across the spirit of what was said rather than the letter? And if we do the latter, what if other participants do not agree with our interpretation? Like Marthe Diepen, I do not have the answer.

Another important issue that emerges from the discussion is the need that the participants felt to discuss issues relating to euthanasia, particularly after having been involved in a case of euthanasia, and the realization that there is no forum in which such matters could be discussed. I frequently noticed this need and saw how the emotional burden of end-of-life decisions weighed on the shoulders of those responsible. It sometimes weighed on my shoulders, and I was only indirectly involved, with no formal responsibility at all. Not only the emotional burden but also the misunderstandings and the interpersonal tensions needed a forum in which they could be expressed. If not brought out into the open, such misunderstandings could remain hidden, though still influencing decisions and actions. The dissatisfaction of the nurses in pulmonology with the way in which, as they saw it, Dr. Glas ignored them when discussing euthanasia with Mrs. Van Nelle and their dissatisfaction with Dr. Glas's "morphine as and when necessary" instructions in the case of Mrs. Lanser are cases in point. The influence of these misunderstandings on the relationships between doctors and nurses on the pulmonology ward continued long after both patients, as individual people, had been forgotten.

A final interesting point that emerges from the discussion is the perception of how frequently euthanasia or euthanasia requests occur. My presence focused attention on euthanasia and seemed to coincide with an increase in its incidence. During my first months at the hospital, this was sometimes the subject of joking, with doctors making remarks such as, "This is the third request this month. Are you sure you're not putting them up to it for your study?" In the previous discussion it is striking that Mieke Van der Ven at first thinks that there have not been many requests for euthanasia in the past few months, only to realize that there had been at least three. This, of course, has serious implications for the reliability of quantitative survey data on the incidence of euthanasia.

Chapter 7

Turning Off Mr. Joost's Respirator

AMYOTROPHIC LATERAL SCLEROSIS

On the evening of July 15, 1992, Mr. Joost, a man of seventy-five, went to the bathroom to remove his dentures before going to bed. When he did not return, his wife went to have a look and found him unconscious on the bathroom floor. She phoned for an ambulance and he was taken to the Randstad Hospital. It soon became clear that he was unable to breathe spontaneously, and he was put on a respirator in intensive care.

Mr. Joost had been unwell for quite some time before his collapse. He had had lung emphysema for years, but lately he had been feeling more tired than usual and was out of breath after even the most minor exertion. Six weeks previously he had fallen down because of a sudden weakness in his leg. Later, both legs started to tremble. His hands also trembled and felt weak, as a result of which he had difficulty grasping things. He had lost weight and his voice had become hoarse.

In the days following his admittance, Mr. Joost remained on the respirator. He was tense and lay sweating and trembling in his bed. He did not sleep and plucked at imaginary things in the air above his bed. After a few such nights, he was given a sedative. In the meantime, various diagnostic tests were carried out. As Mrs. Joost waited tensely for the results, the doctors began to suspect amyotrophic lateral sclerosis (ALS).

I first heard about Mr. Joost when he had been in intensive care for two weeks. Mieke Van der Ven, the anesthetist, called me in the late afternoon of July 28, explained the situation briefly, and asked whether I was interested. I said I was. "It's a problem," she said.

"The man's lungs are not working, but he's there, fully conscious, on the respirator. We've done a whole lot of diagnostic work to find out what's wrong with him. It's probably ALS, and it's going to be a problem. It has nothing to do with euthanasia, but sooner or later, we're going to have to think about stopping treatment of someone who's being kept alive on a respirator."

Attending the doctors' meeting the following morning, I heard that the prognosis was very bad. There were still no definitive results from the tests, but the consensus was that it probably was ALS. Mr. Joost would never be able to breathe independently again, and it would therefore be impossible to wean him from the respirator. Communicating with Mr. Joost was difficult because the tube of the respirator was in his throat, making speech impossible. All Mr. Joost could do was nod or shake his head. He sometimes became restless, even aggressive, and, on several occasions, pulled the respirator tube from his throat.

There was much discussion among the doctors about possible therapies. Mr. Joost could not remain in intensive care indefinitely, and nursing homes catering to patients dependent on a respirator had waiting lists of more than a year. He could have a respirator installed at home, but it was not clear whether Mrs. Joost would be able to cope.

Later that day, Mark Hansen, now ward doctor in intensive care, met with Mr. Joost's family. The relatives had asked for the meeting, and the doctors hoped that they would have thought about the various options.

THE JOOST FAMILY

I attended the meeting together with Mark Hansen and one of the nurses. Mrs. Joost, a small, nervous woman in her sixties, a daughter of about twenty, and a son in his thirties were waiting for us in the coffee lounge. They stood up as we entered, and introductions were made. After everyone was seated again, Mark leaned forward in his chair. "We're now pretty sure that he's got what we call ALS. What this means is that the signals from the nerves in his spine are no longer being transmitted to the lungs. That's why he can't breathe and is dependent on a respirator. It's progressive, which means it will only get worse."

Mark's explanation was followed by many questions from the son and daughter, such as, "So he's never going to get better?" and "So the signals aren't being transmitted properly anymore?" After Mark had spent another half an hour explaining, Mrs. Joost said, wringing her hands nervously, "So, what are the options?"

"Listen," Mark said. "He can't get better. It'll only get worse. He will always be dependent on the respirator."

"So he'll be bedridden?" Mrs. Joost asked.

"Yes, or in a wheelchair."

"Oh," said the son, "so he will be able to move around in a wheelchair?"

"Yes, but he won't be able to go out of the house because he'll always have to be near the machine. He won't be able to take the respirator out of the house. He'll only be able to sit in a chair next to it."

"But what are we going to do?" Mrs. Joost asked, panic rising in her voice. "Will he have to stay in [the] hospital permanently?"

"No, he'll be able to go home, or to a nursing home, and take the respirator with him."

"But I won't be able to manage at home," Mrs. Joost said. "I wouldn't be able to take care of him by myself. He'll have to go to a nursing home."

"That's possible, but there isn't a suitable one here in town."

"Not in town?" Mrs. Joost asked, panic in her voice again.

"No."

A long silence followed. Mrs. Joost sat wringing her hands while concentrating her gaze on the floor in front of her. Then she looked up at Mark. "I don't want to throw him out of the house. You mustn't think that. I'll manage at home. I don't want you to send him to another town."

"His condition will only get worse," Mark repeated. "He will become increasingly dependent until he eventually passes away."

"How long will that take?" asked the daughter.

"I've heard that patients with that disease usually request euthanasia," said the son.

Mrs. Joost looked fiercely at Mark. "I don't want that," she said. "Not active euthanasia."

"No, no, no," said the son, "neither do I, not *active* euthanasia. I'm only saying what I've heard about patients with that illness."

"You don't have to make any decisions now," Mark intervened. "And, in any case, the important thing is what Mr. Joost, himself, wants. We'll have to discuss it with him first."

"But *no* euthanasia," Mrs. Joost repeated.

"No, not euthanasia," the son and daughter said together.

"Yes," Mark said, "but sooner or later we'll have to think about what we're going to do. For example, if he develops pneumonia, then we could treat the pain and shortness of breath, but not the primary infection—"

"I don't want active euthanasia," Mrs. Joost interrupted.

". . . only the pain and shortness of breath in case—"

"Yes, just that."

Later the same day, I heard Mark telling Mieke Van der Ven, the anesthetist, that the Joosts were opposed to active euthanasia, but did not exclude the possibility of passive euthanasia—so they could abstain in case of complications, Mark said. I was surprised when I heard this. It did not seem to me as if Mrs. Joost had agreed to passive euthanasia (i.e., abstention from treating complications), and her interpretation of Mark's last remark and the meaning of her own last remark seemed to me ambiguous, to say the least.

On Friday, July 30, slightly more than two weeks after Mr. Joost had first been admitted to intensive care, the diagnosis of ALS was made official, and the specialists involved (neurologist, pulmonologist, internist, anesthetist, intensive care specialist) concluded that Mr. Joost would now definitely be dependent on the respirator for the rest of his days. The pulmonologist, Dr. Glas, said that he had applied for placement in a suitable nursing home, but it would take a few months at least before one was available. In the meantime, he wanted to optimize Mr. Joost's respiration with a tracheostoma. They decided to consult the psychiatrist to find out whether Mr. Joost was mentally up to this. Serious doubts remained, however, about the feasibility of long-term dependence on the respirator, given the chance of recurrent pneumonia. Mark said that Mr. Joost probably already had nascent pneumonia, and there followed a lengthy discussion as to whether it should be treated.

That afternoon Mark informed Mrs. Joost and her son and daughter of the diagnosis and somber prognosis. Mark said that, sooner or later, a decision would have to be made about what to do in the case of complications, such as pneumonia, for example. Mrs. Joost responded directly and explicitly, "Last time we met we agreed that his life was not to be extended artificially. If he develops pneumonia or any other complication, then he is not to be treated. He must be allowed to die naturally. The situation isn't natural now either, but if we'd have known, then we wouldn't have allowed him to be put on the respirator in the first place. Now he's on it, however, it would be unnatural to turn it off. He wouldn't want that himself either." Mrs. Joost thus confirmed Mark's interpretation of her remarks on the previous Monday.

"Yes," Mark said, "but what if he pulls the tube out himself? It's possible that he might do that to show that he wants it turned off."

"If he pulls it out then it must be replaced," Mrs. Joost said. "He might have pulled it out by accident. We once had an acquaintance who was on a respirator and he pulled out the tube and killed himself. My husband didn't agree with that because it was suicide. So he would never do that to himself. The Lord giveth and the Lord taketh away. He's already on the respirator, so we can't now turn it off, but we mustn't start any new interventions. He must die naturally. There must be *no* helping hand whatsoever."

Mrs. Joost did not want Mark to inform her husband of the diagnosis immediately. She wanted to wait until the tracheostoma had been installed. The following evening she told the nurses that she had informed him of the diagnosis.

In spite of the agreement with Mrs. Joost, the internist and the anesthetist decided during the weekend to treat Mr. Joost's pneumonia with antibiotics. Because they were not 100 percent sure about the prognosis, and given the possibility, however slight, of weaning Mr. Joost from the respirator, they thought that treatment was the safest option. They concluded that they could always abstain from active treatment of complications later when all possible options had been thoroughly investigated.

This decision seemed to be justified on Monday morning when the surgeon who had taken a biopsy questioned the diagnosis of ALS. Some years back, his uncle had come down with similar symptoms and had been diagnosed as having ALS. The uncle had not accepted this and went to another neurologist for a second opinion. The second neurologist found that the symptoms were being caused by the compression of nerves in his back. After a minor operation, the uncle was back to normal. If he had accepted the first diagnosis, he would have been treated as an ALS patient and his back would have remained untreated.

SHIFTING THE BOUNDARY

The problem of treating complications, and even the question of whether Mr. Joost would be able to manage with a respirator at home, now receded into the background, and all attention was directed toward trying to wean him from the respirator. Whether that succeeded or not would determine future policy.

However, when, on Monday afternoon, Mrs. Joost heard that her husband had been given antibiotics during the weekend and that the doctors were now seriously investigating the possibility of weaning him from the respirator, she was furious. She said to one of the nurses, in a high-pitched, irritated voice, "The agreement was that nothing would be done to artificially extend his life, and that no attempt would be made to wean him from the machine. That's how we interpreted the conclusions of the meeting on Friday. We've had the children round and the grandchildren have said their good-byes. Everybody was resigned to the situation, and now this is being disrupted." She was also angry that Gerrit Knol, who had replaced Mark Hansen as junior doctor on intensive care, had discussed the prognosis with her husband.

That afternoon, a second neurologist (the first one had gone on leave) confirmed the ALS diagnosis, thereby putting an end to the doubt and speculation. He also managed to calm Mrs. Joost, had a long talk with Mr. Joost, and reinstated the agreement to not actively treat complications. He discussed the tracheostoma with Mr. Joost, and it was agreed that this would go ahead because it would increase his comfort. Otherwise, the only interventions would be the removal of mucus from his lungs, treatment of possible bleeding after the tracheostoma had been inserted, and the use of morphine in case of shortness of breath.

A few days later, on Thursday, August 5, I had a discussion with Harry Post, one of the intensive care (IC) nurses. "The Lord giveth and the Lord taketh away," he said with a sigh. "That's a recurring theme, you know: that they won't tolerate any helping hand. And the doctors are respecting it. They've agreed to stop with the antibiotics. But they haven't said a word about the other medication, or the food. In connection with the respirator they say, 'That was already installed, so we have to leave it as it is.' But then what about the tracheostoma? Isn't that an intervention? And they've said, 'Nothing that will extend his life artificially.' But if you keep feeding him through a tube, isn't that extending his life artificially? Where do you draw the line? And take the tracheostoma. If there's bleeding, what will they do? They'll have to treat it. 'Yes,' they say, '*those* are complications we have to treat.' When the relatives start thinking about that, it's quite likely that they'll come to the nurses with awkward questions."

"What strikes me," I said, "is that nobody seems to bother asking Mr. Joost what he wants."

"The new neurologist has talked to him," Harry said. "He's discussed everything with him."

"Did he tell him that they were going to abstain from actively treating complications and that he would probably die sooner because of that?"

"Yes, well, what do we mean by abstinence?"

"I mean that they won't treat opportunistic infections."

"I don't know exactly what he told him. I wasn't there."

"It seems to me that his wife is making all the decisions, when he is quite capable of making them himself. Is that the way things are usually done here?"

Harry was silent.

"What strikes me," I said after a while, "is how much emphasis is always placed on the patient's right of self-determination. What the relatives think is always secondary. But here, all of a sudden, it's the other way round."

"Yes, well, the communication with the patient isn't optimal here, is it? So one has to depend on what the relatives say. There hasn't been much attempt to talk to him, actually."

"And why not?" I asked. "Is it that they haven't bothered because it's difficult, or is it that they think his wife is communicating what he really wants? What do you think?"

"The idea was to try and find out what the relatives thought first. Usually it isn't possible to communicate adequately with IC patients, so you *have* to discuss [the situation] with the relatives. It's not often that you have IC patients on the respirator who are fully conscious and able to communicate adequately."

"Do you think he'll die on the weekend?"

"No, I don't think so. It could take a long time yet."

"It *could* take a long time, but *will* it take a long time?"

"Depends on the patient."

"So he'll probably be here for a long time?"

"Yes, unless he gets a real complication. And we *are* provoking complications."

"What do you mean?"

"Well, we've stopped the tube feeding, and most of the medication, et cetera, so you can expect pneumonia anytime."

At that moment, Jan, another nurse, came in. He said that Mrs. Joost had not been aware that the nasogastric feeding had been stopped. He said he had been talking to her and she had asked whether her husband was getting fluids. Jan had answered that he was. She then asked, "He is being fed, isn't he?" "No," Jan answered. "Oh," said Mrs. Joost, and walked away.

The following day, the internist had an appointment with Mrs. Joost to explain that the tube feeding had been stopped. Mrs. Joost cancelled the appointment, saying that she had to go somewhere and did not *really* need to speak to the doctor. It was quite clear what the arrangement was; she said, "Not to keep him alive artificially, but not to pull out the plug either." When Mr. Joost's son left the hospital half an hour later, he said, "What an agony. Maybe it would have been better to pull out the plug." Mr. Joost was now looking much worse, with sunken cheeks and dark rings around his eyes.

When I arrived on the intensive care ward on Monday morning, August 9, Mr. Joost had just been wheeled into the [surgical] theater for the installation of the tracheostoma. A group of nurses were having a discussion in the corridor.

"Would the decision have been different if there'd been a place available in a nursing home?" Jan asked Harry.

"I doubt it," Harry answered. "It would have been exactly the same, except we would have been rid of him sooner and they would have had the problem."

"They've stopped all medication and the tube feeding," said Elizabeth.

"Yes," Jan said. "But what's the difference between pulling the plug or giving him a jab now and letting him die of starvation in a couple of weeks?"

"The difference lies in the duration," Harry said. "It's less radical, but there's no real qualitative difference."

"Mrs. Joost said that if he pulls out the tube then it has to be replaced; otherwise, it would be suicide," Elizabeth said.

"Ach," said Harry, "she's much too fond of talking for him."

"It seems as though he might be here for weeks yet," I said.

"No, that won't happen," said Harry.

"Oh?" I said.

"Yes," Harry said. "The idea is not to intervene if he extubates himself, for example. If he pulls that thing out and we don't get there in time, then that'll be that. He's on thirty percent oxygen at the moment. If things have to be natural, then they should alter that as well."

Ironically, however, after that afternoon, the notes in the nursing records became increasingly optimistic:

> Seems cheerful. Has been trying to eat some soup himself. If the situation continues to improve then it seems desirable to investigate the possibility of a place in a nursing home.

That evening someone added:

> Eaten some soup. Had a reasonable evening. Wife's birthday. They celebrated. Now has a typewriter with which to communicate.

The following morning, Mr. Joost actually got out of bed to wash his hair, albeit with much assistance from the nurses.

On the morning of Wednesday, August 11, I accompanied Dr. Glas to see Mr. Joost. He looked a lot better than the last time I had seen him. He was wide awake and clear-eyed. He was able to communicate voicelessly and we had a short conversation.

That afternoon the case notes were somber:

> No chance of a place in a suitable nursing home, and arrangements for respiration at home would take so long that the patient would have probably died by the time things were ready. Conclusion: we must assume that he will be here up until the end.

This was repeated in the nursing records, with the addition "Euthanasia is not an option."

On Friday, August 13, the specialists involved in Mr. Joost's case had a long discussion about the continuation of respiration and the line through which Mr. Joost was still receiving fluid.

TURNING OFF THE RESPIRATOR

On Monday, August 16, a decision was made to stop the administration of fluid through an intravenous drip because this was an "unnatural" intervention and gradually to reduce the oxygen until it was down to a normal 21 percent. Possible complications were to be treated with morphine. Only the enemas would be continued (Mr. Joost was constipated) because this was symptomatic. That evening the neurologist discussed the decision with Mr. Joost, who agreed. The following morning the neurologist informed Mrs. Joost, who nodded, but said nothing.

On Friday, August 20, I had a discussion with Gerrit Knol, the IC junior doctor. I asked him why they had now decided to stop the fluid and reduce the oxygen.

"Don't ask me," he said, shrugging. "The reasons are not clear to me yet either. I don't agree with what's happening. On Friday, they suddenly decided—it was the anesthetist's idea—that if it was going to be natural, as the relatives wanted it to be—which I really don't understand either—then he should be on twenty-one percent oxygen. The reasoning was that *if* he was to go to a nursing home, then he would have to be on twenty-one percent oxygen anyway. It was a practical reason. But, in the meantime, the decision had been made that he wouldn't be leaving the hospital at all. So what's the reason for reducing it? I think it's in order to speed things up a bit. One of the anesthetists wanted to reduce it on Friday, but I resisted because if he'd died then it would really have been euthanasia. He didn't agree."

"Why were you opposed?"

"Look, I also think this is an agony for the man, and I don't agree with what his relatives want, but we have to respect it, I think. But it's a bit ambiguous because we weren't giving him food, and now we've stopped the fluid as well. So it's gradually being shut down. He's already told his wife that he thought the acquaintance who extubated himself had committed suicide, so he was obviously opposed to that sort of thing. So if they're carrying out a kind of veiled euthanasia then it's just not fair. And they hadn't discussed it with the relatives, that's why I was opposed. The neurologist had the impression that the relatives didn't want to be told too much, that they didn't want to make too many decisions themselves. And now there's a new IC specialist, Emiel."

Later that afternoon I went to IC to see if there were any new developments. One of the nurses on duty said that nothing much had happened. There were signs of a nascent pneumonia. "Which we won't treat," he added. That evening one of the nurses wrote:

Eating and drinking himself. Oxygen reduced to 21 percent.

On the weekend the report read as follows:

In a good mood. Feet and legs very edematous. Values the small things in life, like good food.

In the nursing records on Tuesday, August 24, I read "LOTS OF PURULENT SPUTUM. Patient calm." Later that day one of the nurses reported this to the doctors during a staff meeting. "Well, we are waiting for a complication, aren't we?" Gerrit said, cynically, only to add immediately, "No, I didn't mean that. That wasn't a very nice thing to say."

"Yes," said the anesthetist, "but it *is* true; let's be honest." Everyone was silent.

During the following days Mr. Joost continued to eat and drink well. The nurses arranged for the nutritionist to make a special menu for him, with his favorite dishes. The logopedist had installed an apparatus to improve communication. During the day he practiced, and in the evenings he watched television. He was still producing a lot of sputum.

On the weekend of August 28 and 29, Mr. Joost's condition deteriorated considerably. He said he felt weak and short of breath. The bedsores on his back had become much larger, and he could now only lie on his side.

On Monday, August 30, I went to the IC ward to see if anything was happening. In the corridor I encountered Harry, and we started chatting. I was telling him something when I noticed he was not listening. He held his head slightly to one side and seemed to be concentrating on some sound in the distance. I stopped talking and listened. A beeping sound was barely audible. Our eyes met.

"That's Mr. Joost's respirator," he said. "It must have got disconnected." He stood listening for a few more seconds. "We'd better go and have a look, hadn't we? Otherwise, things might become unpleasant for the fellow." He moved off in the direction of Mr. Joost's room. I followed. Mr. Joost was propped up with two large pillows. His head was partly turned to one side. One eye was closed and the other half open, with only the white showing. I thought he was dead. The respirator pipe was resting loosely on his chest, and the machine was issuing nervous beeps.

"You're not connected to the machine," Harry said. "Shall we reconnect you again then?" He pushed the end of the pipe back into the tracheostoma in Mr. Joost's throat. After a few seconds, Mr. Joost opened his eye and both eyes slowly turned back to their normal position. He was awake.

"Well, the respirator was disconnected. How did that happen?" Harry asked, and after a few seconds of silence, "Are you okay now?"

At that moment Jan, another nurse, came in.

"The respirator was disconnected," Harry said.

"You weren't trying to test us, were you?" Jan asked.

"It took two minutes," Harry said, looking sternly at his watch.

"You mean you stood there listening for two minutes first?" Jan asked.

"Yes, two minutes. He could have been dead."

"Yes, he could have been dead."

The three of us walked away.

"Is it likely that something like that could happen and you don't hear the alarm?" I asked.

"Yes," Jan said, "especially if the volume is turned down, or turned off. In that case, it would be quite likely that if the tube came loose, we wouldn't notice."

"Do you ever turn the volume down?" I asked.

Harry gave me a meaningful glance and said nothing.

"Can the tube come off easily, just like that?"

"Yes, it *has* to come off easily. We have to remove it to be able to suck the sputum from his lungs," Harry said.

The records on Wednesday, September 2, read as follows:

> Weak, losing weight rapidly. Becoming less lively. Is resigned to the situation. Seems to be developing a fever. Sucked up lots of sputum.

Nine days later, on September 11, the records read:

> Deteriorating rapidly. Hardly drinking anything. Becoming increasingly drowsy. Hardly reacts when spoken to. Tense, fingers grasping nervously. 10 mg morphine i.v.

On Sunday, September 13, one of the nurses had written the following:

> We were all in the coffee lounge discussing Mr. Joost. He's stopped eating and drinking. He's just lying there, dehydrating and becoming edematous. Bedsores spreading. Wasting away. Doesn't want morphine. When you ask him whether he's in pain, he shakes his head. That's just about all he can do. The only unnatural thing now is the machine, which is going to draw out the dying process. Can we, the nurses, go on like this? What are we going to do with similar cases in the future? Dr. Alders [one of the anesthetists] came by and asked how

things were going. I said that things could continue like this for ages, as long as the machine was there. She then altered the setting (gave instructions to).

The next evening Mr. Joost died. The following morning I spoke to Harry.

"I hear Mr. Joost has died." I said.

"Yes."

"What happened?"

"His heart," Harry said, as he beat rapidly against his chest with palm of his hand and raised his eyebrows in a manner that I interpreted as cynical.

"His heart?"

"Yes."

"I suppose it was to be expected, given he was no longer eating and drinking."

"Yes, definitely."

WHAT THE NURSES SAID, AND WHAT THEY MEANT

I never found out what really happened during Mr. Joost's final hours, although the statements of some of the nurses were very suggestive. When I suggested to Harry that Mr. Joost might be in the hospital for weeks to come, he answered, "No, that won't happen . . . the idea is not to intervene if he extubates himself." However, when, some time later, I was talking to Harry in the corridor and the alarm on Mr. Joost's respirator went off, Harry restored the connection. I do not think that the fact that he did not rush to Mr. Joost's bedside and do this as soon as he heard the alarm can be interpreted as an attempt to let Mr. Joost die. If this had been the nurses' intention, then they certainly would not have done so in the presence of a researcher with a tape recorder in his hand. And, if they only reconnected the tube because I was watching, then there was no need to wait that long before doing so. After all, Harry had heard the alarm beeping right from the start. Moreover, we may assume that Harry knew exactly how much time he had to reconnect the tube from the moment that he first heard the alarm. What was happening here was probably a bit of social drama, enacted partly for my benefit and partly for each other (hence the scene at the bedside), rather than an attempt to let Mr. Joost die. If Harry had wanted the latter, all he had to do was ignore the alarm. It must have been obvious to him that I had not heard it, and by cocking his head so emphatically, he drew my attention to the sound.

The extreme statements by some of the nurses should not be interpreted as a literal expression of what they thought, but rather as an expression of the tension and frustration after two months of uncertainty (see the entry in the nursing records on September 13). The nurses' discourse was also a product of the tensions and rivalries inherent in the relationship between themselves and the doctors. The specialists might have known a patient for years from regular visits to their outpatient clinic, whereas the nurses only see the patient during his or her stay in the hospital. On the other hand, during that stay, the doctor might only make a couple of brief visits during a week, while the nurses are involved, often intimately, with the patient twenty-four hours a day. Both can claim to know what the patient "really" wants and what is good for him or her, but the doctor, because of his or her rank, status, and training, decides policy. These tensions are inherent in the doctor-nurse relationship, generally, but they are more extreme in intensive care. Intensive care nurses are the specialists among the nurses. Experienced IC nurses often know more than young, inexperienced junior doctors, but the latter still have more influence on policy.

In the case of Mr. Joost, the nurses formed a relatively tight group with shared ideas. The doctors were much less homogenous as a group. These differences were exacerbated by the different specializations and the rapid alternation of doctors, each having a different style and different ideas. During the weekly IC meetings there were always different faces among the doctors, whereas Harry and Jan were always present to represent the nurses.

DOUBT, UNCERTAINTY, AND HESITATION

Mr. Joost's case was complex, and many shifts in policy occurred during his two-month stay in intensive care. Decisions were made, repealed, and reinstated. Specialists alternated rapidly, and many hours were spent discussing what to do. When Mr. Joost was first admitted, the doctors suspected ALS. After a first series of diagnostic tests, the neurologist confirmed this diagnosis. Later it was questioned by the surgeon but then reconfirmed by a second neurologist. The frequent changes in policy relating to the possibility of weaning Mr. Joost from the respirator were related to the uncertain diagnosis.

Some of the doubt and hesitation was a result of the frequent alternation of specialists involved in the case. This was due to various factors. First, the complicated nature of Mr. Joost's illness demanded the participation of specialists from different disciplines. Second, because he had been in the hospital so long, he had experienced the routine circulation of junior doctors within the department of internal medicine. Third, it was summer, and many of the doctors went on leave, thus further increasing the frequency of alternation. As a result, four junior doctors, three anesthetists, two surgeons, two neurologists, one pulmonologist, one psychiatrist, and a whole host of nurses working in three shifts, to say nothing of the doctors on night and weekend duty, had been involved in the case.

The uncertainty was further increased by the custom of reifying the various categories of personnel and the different medical specializations. In discussions, the participants did not talk about Harry and Jan, or Dr. Roelofs and Dr. Glas; rather, they talked about "the nurses," "internal medicine," "pulmonology," neurology," and so on. Groups of individuals were collectivized, and as a result, all the individual differences were glossed over in the formal discourse of the written case notes and the meetings to discuss policy. All that remained of complex differences of opinion was, "the nurses are dissatisfied," "neurology thinks this," "internal wants that."

Different disciplinary approaches and related insights into aspects of Mr. Joost's illness, and differences in personality and experience, led to diverging opinions and ways of doing things. This was clearly visible in the case of the two neurologists. The first neurologist did not bother to talk with Mr. Joost and assumed that Mrs. Joost was an acceptable representative. This neurologist became uneasy whenever even the remote possibility of euthanasia arose, and this may explain his avoidance of direct communication with Mr. Joost. The second neurologist did not avoid difficult end-of-life decisions and went straight to Mr. Joost to discuss the matter.

The doubt and hesitation were also related to the ambiguous nature of the concept of abstention. Did it include nasogastric feeding, or fluid through an intravenous drip? What of symptomatic interventions such as sucking the sputum from the lungs or using enemas in case of constipation? Where did abstention from treating complications end, and where did palliative symptomatic treatment begin?

Recent history was also important. Just before I started my study, Dr. Glas had had an emphysema patient, Mr. Leenders, in intensive care. He was on a respirator and had a similar condition and prognosis to Mr. Joost. One day Mr. Leenders asked Dr. Glas to turn off the respirator so that he could die. After long discussions with Mr. Leenders, he agreed. Dr. Glas was not sure whether this was euthanasia or not, so he reported it as euthanasia to the public prosecutor. Although it clearly was *not* euthanasia (a patient has the *right* to refuse treatment, and the doctor is obliged to respect this), the public prosecutor ordered an investigation. The investigation concluded that no offense had been committed, but the inconvenience caused (Dr. Glas only knew for certain that he would not be prosecuted more than a year after he reported the incident) definitely left its mark on the hospital. Mr. Leenders was mentioned countless times during discussions about Mr. Joost. If a criminal investigation could be instigated for simply respecting a patient's rights, what would the consequences be in the more ambiguous case of a decision to hasten death?

Another important reason for the doubt and hesitation was the presence of two conflicting motivations among the doctors. On the one hand, they had a fundamental aversion toward hastening the death of a patient who had not explicitly requested it (which is why they treated Mr. Joost's pneumonia during his first weekend on the intensive care ward, contrary to the agreed-upon policy and the wishes of the relatives), and on the other hand, they realized that if they allowed opportunistic infections to go untreated while alleviating symptoms, then they would release Mr. Joost from suffering.

The case was further complicated by the inadequate communication with Mr. Joost. Initially this was because they *could* not communicate with him. Later, however, even though the tracheostoma made communication possible and the second neurologist and various other specialists talked to him, the doctors still tended to rely on Mrs. Joost for their information about what Mr. Joost wanted. Because patients in intensive care are usually unconscious, a specific pattern of communication developed in which the relatives rather than the patients, were central, and this pattern was maintained even when it was not necessary.

The shifting definition of what was "natural" and the increasingly implicit nature of communication with Mrs. Joost were also important. The dying process was to be as "natural" as possible, that is with as little medical intervention as possible. "Unnatural" interventions that had already occurred (putting him on the respirator) were to be maintained because they had become the "natural" situation, but no new interventions were to be initiated, and opportunistic infections and complications were to go untreated. However, exactly what was natural and unnatural tended to shift, and the line between them was quite arbitrary. As the definitions shifted and more and more "unnatural" interventions were terminated, Mrs. Joost's communication became increasingly implicit. Her message was "Abstain as much as possible but I don't want to be told explicitly."

Mr. Joost's physical condition also shifted. At one point, the situation seemed to be clear: the diagnosis was confirmed; Mr. Joost would have to remain in the hospital because his wife could not take care of him at home and there were no beds available in suitable nursing homes; the family had accepted the situation and was already in a process of anticipatory mourning; and policy was starting to focus consistently on letting the patient die by abstaining from treating complications and gradually reducing the nasogastric feeding and fluids. By that time, Mr. Joost could communicate adequately, and he made it known that he agreed with this policy. However, at the same time, it seemed as though he was starting to fight back, physically. When the tube feeding was finally stopped, Mr. Joost started, with increasing appetite, to eat on his own, and when the intravenous fluids were turned off, Mr. Joost resumed drinking independently. This revival was short-lived, but it tended to raise new questions and doubts regarding abstention.

The decisions that crystallized were therefore influenced by a great many factors, both medical and nonmedical: the difficult diagnosis and prognosis, the absence of a place in a nursing home, the length of Mr. Joost's stay in intensive care (and the fact that it was intensive care), the large number of different specialists involved in his treatment, the shifting boundaries of what was considered natural, ambiguity of the concept of abstinence, the initial difficulty in communicating with the patient, the professional relationship between specialists and nurses, and, finally, the individual personalities and experiences of those involved.

Chapter 8

When Doctors Refuse
a Euthanasia Request

MR. OOSTEN'S EUTHANASIA REQUEST

Weekly Rounds, January, 1993

We were in the room of two elderly male patients. Dr. Schuyt and Dr. Glas, the ward doctor, and a medical student were busy with the patient by the window. They had pulled the curtain closed around his bed and were bunched together, maneuvering about so that they could take turns listening to his lungs through a stethoscope. As it was too crowded around the bed, I was standing on the opposite side of the room and could see only feet and moving shapes outlined in the curtain.

In the other bed lay an old man with a half-moon profile: high forehead, pointed chin, long hooked nose, and a mouth that had caved in, in the absence of supporting dentures. He mumbled something about his treatment, that I didn't understand. He looked at me intensely through dark, beady eyes. I thought that maybe he was senile and said that he had better wait for the doctors, that they would be with him in a moment, as soon as they had finished with his neighbor. On the wall opposite his bed hung a small oil painting of a lake surrounded by mountains. The colors were dark, which gave the impression of age. The style was dated, but at the same time, there was something modern about it. I walked over to have a closer look.

"My mother painted that. She was an artist," he said, in a voice that was suddenly forceful and clear. I turned around, but at that moment, Dr. Schuyt emerged from the curtain and came over to Mr. Oosten's bed. From their exchange, I gathered that Mr. Oosten had been admitted because of impaired breathing as a result of terminal pulmonary emphysema. Dr. Schuyt said that they could not do much for him in the hospital and that he would submit an application for admittance to a nursing home. Mr. Oosten sighed and said nothing.

Weekly Rounds, January 19

Two weeks later, a new ward doctor, Albert Meertens, arrived. Before rounds, Dr. Glas spent half an hour going through the case notes of all the patients on the ward with him. They came to Mr. Oosten.

"That's someone who wants euthanasia," Dr. Glas said, as he looked around at me. "Weren't you here last Monday during rounds?"

"No," I answered.

"He asked for euthanasia. I didn't consider the request relevant, but I agreed that we would abstain if he contracted pneumonia. I've discussed it with his daughter. He's an old COPD patient. He's waiting for a place in a nursing home."

After that we did the rounds: Dr. Glas, Albert, Connie (one of the nurses), and me. Dr. Schuyt was on vacation. At one point, Dr. Glas and Albert were examining a patient, while Connie and I stood outside in the corridor, leaning on the trolley containing the patients' case notes.

"Mr. Oosten is an interesting case for you," she said. "He keeps asking for euthanasia."

"I know," I said. "Glas just told me that he requested it last Monday during rounds."

"Not only then," she said. "He keeps imploring the doctors for euthanasia, and not only them but the nurses and anyone else who happens to be around as well. He's got a euthanasia declaration and everything, but they just won't listen to him. He's actually Schuyt's patient, but he never comes to see him; he hasn't even spoken to him."

I was just about to say that I wondered whether he would broach the topic of euthanasia again this morning and how Dr. Glas would react, when a loud, nervous bleep, bleep, bleep became audible.

"My beeper," Dr. Glas called, and rushed past us in search of a telephone. A few minutes later he returned to say that he had to leave to perform a bronchoscopy and that Albert would finish the rounds.

An hour later, when it was finally Mr. Oosten's turn, Albert looked at his watch and clapped his hands.

"Right," he said, "it's one o'clock, time for lunch."

When, later in the afternoon, we finally came to Mr. Oosten's bedside, he appeared introverted and didn't say anything at all.

Weekly Rounds, January 26

Before rounds, Dr. Glas and Albert discussed the patients. Dr. Schuyt was still on vacation. They went through all the patients systematically. When they got to Mr. Oosten, Dr. Glas put his file aside.

"Well," he said, "at least we don't need to say anything about him. It's a clear case."

I had been waiting for them to discuss Mr. Oosten's case.

"Why won't you grant his request for euthanasia? It's clear and consistent, isn't it?" I asked.

"Yes, but he's not yet in the terminal phase," Dr. Glas replied.

"Neither was Mrs. Van Nelle," I said, somewhat provocatively.

"Yes, but that was a *completely* different case," Dr. Glas said, leaning back in his chair. "Hers was a case of unbearable suffering. Mr. Oosten is not really in *such* bad condition. He's not suffering like Mrs. Van Nelle. When you look at him lying there in bed, you get the impression that his condition is bearable. His real problem is that he doesn't want to go to a nursing home."

I asked Dr. Glas if he would introduce me to Mr. Oosten formally; then it would be easier for me to discuss his euthanasia request with him. Dr. Glas thought this was a good idea.

During rounds, we discovered that Mr. Oosten had been moved to another room, which he shared with a patient whom Connie said was "far gone."

"This is Dr. Meertens, the new ward doctor," Dr. Glas said as we entered, forgetting that Albert had been doing the daily rounds for the past two weeks.

"Who?" Mr. Oosten asked, screwing up his face.

"Dr. Meertens, the ward doctor."

Albert shook his hand anyway.

"How are you doing?" Dr. Glas asked.

Mr. Oosten said that he was short of breath, but that was not what occupied his thoughts. He had a whole list of complaints, and he took the time to enumerate them. He articulated each word separately, as though he was learning some new and difficult language from a book.

"I . . . don't . . . like . . . this . . . new . . . room," he said. "Take . . . that . . . cupboard . . . there . . . for . . . example." He pointed to the steel cupboard that stood between his bed and the window rather than in its usual place between his bed and that of his neighbor.

"It's . . . between . . . my . . . bed . . . and . . . the . . . window . . . Now . . . I . . . can't . . . put . . . anything . . . on . . . the . . . windowsill."

Dr. Glas turned to Connie. "Why can't he have his cupboard on the other side?"

"That's okay with me," she said, shrugging. "But when it's there, his neighbor uses it to store his urine samples, and Mr. Oosten doesn't like that either, does he?" She looked critically at Mr. Oosten, who looked back innocently.

Through the thick bandages covering his lower lip and chin, the neighbor said, "Well, if it will be of any help. . . ."

"Yes, well, maybe we can try again," Dr. Glas said.

"Please do," Mr. Oosten said, and laid his head back on his pillow with a sigh of satisfaction, only to resume his list of complaints.

"Then there's the other issue I want to discuss with you: euthanasia. I want euthanasia. I've mentioned this before. I don't want to go on like this. It is hopeless and I want you to put an end to it. I want euthanasia." He spoke slowly, in a quiet voice, and when he used the word euthanasia, he emphasized each syllable: eu-tha-na-sia. It seemed as though he thought that Dr. Glas would not understand otherwise.

"Are you having much pain, or are you short of breath?" Dr. Glas asked.

"I want eu-tha-na-sia."

"Yes, maybe you're right, but it's not something that we can just carry out on demand." He turned to me. "That's why I want to introduce you to Dr. Pool. He's a lawyer . . . no . . . he's an an-thro-pol-o-gist. . . ."

"Anthropology . . . the science of man?" Mr. Oosten said, raising his eyebrows.

Dr. Glas beamed. "Precisely, he's a *medical* anthropologist, and he's doing research on the very topic you were talking about. . . ."

"Eu-tha-na-sia."

"Exactly. It might be a good idea if you discussed it with him. Maybe it would clarify the whole issue. Is it all right if he comes along and talks to you?"

"What?"

"Is it okay if Dr. Pool comes and discusses your euthanasia request with you?"

"Yes, yes."

"Good."

We moved on to the next patient.

Later on, when we were alone in the doctors' office, I said to Albert that I wondered why Dr. Glas seemed to ignore Mr. Oosten's euthanasia request. Albert said that he was also surprised. If it were up to him, he would grant it, he said. He did not think that it was justified simply to assume that Mr. Oosten was not suffering as unbearably as he said he was. He said that he had discussed the matter with Dr. Glas, but that Dr. Glas had explained that he didn't want to interfere with one of Dr. Schuyt's patients while he was away on vacation.

Daily Rounds, January 27

The following day, I accompanied Albert during his daily rounds. When we reached Mr. Oosten, Albert asked him how he felt.

"Who are you?" Mr. Oosten asked suspiciously.

"Albert Meertens, the ward doctor," he answered.

"Who?"

"The ward doctor."

"Oh."

He looked at me suspiciously, and I did not get the impression that he recognized me. My initial suspicion that he might be suffering from senile dementia surfaced again. I might have to be introduced all over again.

Later in the afternoon I went to see him anyway.

"You're the an-thro-pol-o-gist" he said, when I asked him if he remembered me. He was still willing to discuss his euthanasia request with me but asked if we could do it the next day, as he felt tired and wanted to rest. I promised to visit the next afternoon.

MR. OOSTEN'S DEATH

The next morning, Mr. Oosten became acutely short of breath. He gasped and struggled for air. He was moved to a separate room. Albert telephoned Dr. Glas and asked if he could prescribe morphine. Dr. Glas agreed. Later, during the afternoon, his condition appeared to improve, but I decided not to bother him with my interview. In the early evening, his condition deteriorated again. His sister arrived and started to pressure Albert to give him "a shot." Albert thought it unnecessary to trouble Dr. Glas at home about administering morphine, given the situation was the same as in the morning. He gave Mr. Oosten 5 mg of morphine. Mr. Oosten died a few hours later.

"So euthanasia wasn't necessary after all?" I asked, when I saw Albert the next morning.

He looked at me for a long time but didn't say anything.

"It wasn't euthanasia, was it?" I asked.

"Not euthanasia? Well, actually . . ." He fell silent and stared out the window.

THE NURSING RECORDS

After Mr. Oosten's death, I read through the reports that the nursing staff had kept of his condition and treatment.

December 26

Was brought to the ward on a stretcher at 10:30. Accompanied by his daughter. Was short of breath, seemed to panic occasionally.

Reason for admittance: shortness of breath. Is immobile because of seriously impaired breathing as a result of terminal pulmonary emphysema.

Religion: Catholic, but doesn't go to church, etc.

Lives by himself. Two daughters. District nurse washes him, makes sandwiches, etc.; daughters do the shopping, etc.

Wife died six months ago. Since then has nothing more to live for.

Joined a "euthanasia club" [the Association for Voluntary Euthanasia]—euthanasia declaration in his drawer.

Mental ability, orientation, hygiene, etc., all good.

A bit deaf, no pain, but short of breath.

DNR

[Many pages were devoted to the patient's shortness of breath and bowel movement, during the period from December 26 until January 11.]

January 11

Very short of breath this morning. Longs for death but is scared of suffocating . . .

January 12

Short of breath when he moves.

Says that he would like to die soon. Doesn't want to go to a nursing home, but realizes that he has no choice.

Discussed his euthanasia request with Dr. Glas. Won't grant his request, but has discussed limits to treatment: hopeless complications won't be treated.

Dr. Schuyt must arrange DNR order.

January 13

Get Dr. Schuyt to arrange DNR order.

January 14

DNR order still has to be arranged. Hasn't been done yet.

Was looked after, didn't have the energy to do anything himself. Really wants to die. Has only one wish, and that is euthanasia. Has discussed this with the doctor. Is very scared of suffocating. Was short of breath again this evening.

January 15

DNR?

Expressed the desire for euthanasia again this morning. Very clear!!!!!
Wants to see the doctor in connection with euthanasia request.
Rounds: ward doctor to discuss euthanasia request with specialist.
Expressed the desire to die again.
Daughter visited.

January 16

Hardly slept. Was in a good mood.
Schuyt still has to see patient. He is looking forward to meeting.
Sleeps a lot; seems to have changed day/night rhythm around.

January 18

Had a moderate day. Complains constantly of shortness of breath.
Sat in his chair the whole morning.
Try to arrange a meeting with Dr. Schuyt tomorrow morning about his euthanasia request.
Is continually short of breath.

January 19

Didn't sleep all that well.
Arrange euthanasia discussion today.
Gets tired and short of breath quickly. Everything is too much for him. Would like to see more action with regard to his euthanasia request.
No appointment with Schuyt yet.

January 20

Last night shorter of breath than usual. Was awake the whole night. Hopes that he will see Schuyt today. Is worried that he is not being taken seriously.
Arrange an appointment with daughters to discuss the future. *Absolutely* opposed to admittance to a nursing home.

January 21

Appointment Albert and daughters.

January 22

Demanded the necessary attention. Other than that, not a spectacular night.
Still short of breath, but realizes that it won't improve.

January 23

Calm night.
Didn't complain much about shortness of breath.

January 25

Calm night, only rang the bell once.
Says he can't get enough air.
Still short of breath . . .

January 26

Rings bell continually without clear reason. Is demanding.
Please evaluate euthanasia request.
Dr. Schuyt is still on vacation. Euthanasia request has still not been evaluated. He mentioned it again himself.
Knows what his end will be like. Dr. Pool will discuss euthanasia with him.
Complained about the position of his cupboard. Has been explained a number of times. Apart from that, calm.

January 27

Evaluation of euthanasia discussion with Dr. Pool?
Everything the same as usual.
Is scared.
Bell wasn't working.

January 28

Has serious bedsores.
Condition suddenly deteriorated at 15:30. Was moved to another
room. Daughters have been alerted and are present.
Later some improvement.
May receive 5 mg of morphine. Is aware of this.
Felt better; wasn't bothered too much by shortness of breath
(warn daughters in case of morphine).
Restless since 20:00. Short of breath.
Was given 5 mg of morphine s.c. [subcutaneous] in consultation
with Albert.

20:25—passed away.

THE DOCTORS' INTERPRETATIONS

Albert Meertens

The day after Mr. Oosten died, Albert went on vacation. One
morning shortly after his return, three weeks later, we were sitting
in the doctors' office drinking coffee. One of the doctors was having one of those rare moments when he had nothing pressing to do.
He even asked me whether I wanted to ask him any questions.
"Yes," I said. "When Mr. Oosten died, just before you went on
vacation, I asked you whether it had been euthanasia. You didn't
answer, but I had the impression that you thought it might have
been. Was it?"
"No, it wasn't, really, but we did . . . let me see. . . . If you decide
to abstain from treating someone in his condition, and you only give

them morphine to alleviate shortness of breath, then that isn't euthanasia because we don't call it euthanasia. You know that he is going
to die, but it isn't euthanasia, no."

"So the primary intention was alleviating his shortness of breath?" I
asked.

"Okay, but in the case of someone with that degree of pulmonary
disease, you know that if you alleviate his shortness of breath then
he will stop breathing altogether. You *know* that beforehand."

"Can't you just give enough morphine to alleviate the shortness
of breath, but without letting him die?"

"No, that won't work. It's impossible because that shortness of
breath is the very reason that he keeps on breathing. If you alleviate
his shortness of breath, then he simply stops breathing altogether."

"So if a patient in that condition requests euthanasia, then, in
theory, you can always grant that request unofficially by simply
alleviating his shortness of breath with morphine?"

"If you set the condition for yourself that you *really* think that he
experiences his shortness of breath as unbearable, then yes. But
otherwise, in the condition that Mr. Oosten was in at the beginning,
no. In that case shortness of breath is unpleasant but it doesn't lead
to acute fear of suffocating. When he was first admitted, Mr. Oosten
slept at night without fear, but at the end, he was nothing *but* short
of breath. And, in any case, he would probably have died without
morphine anyway."

"Was he becoming senile or was he just . . .? I sometimes had the
impression that he was senile, but according to the nurses, he was
quite lucid."

"He wasn't senile."

"I sometimes had the impression he didn't know who it was he was
talking to, and he kept forgetting who everyone was, and . . .."

"I think . . . his CO_2 was very high, and one of the consequences
of that is that the brain doesn't function properly. He was also old,
and old people tend to forget things. That isn't senility. He knew
exactly what he wanted and what he didn't want, and he could
discuss it lucidly."

"So you could take his repeated requests for euthanasia seriously?"

"Yes, yes. He certainly wasn't senile in the sense there was reason to doubt that his request was serious."

"So why do you think it wasn't granted?"

"I think it was because he was in relatively good condition. . . Well, good condition, acceptable condition . . . as a doctor you must, I think, draw a line between what is acceptable suffering and what isn't. I don't know what I would have decided if I had been responsible for making the decision."

"You also mentioned something about his sister."

"Yes, when I went into his room, his sister was there, and . . . she took my hand and said, 'Doctor, Doctor, give him a shot quickly; otherwise, it's going to take too long.' That kind of thing makes me sick. When I hear something like that I feel like saying, 'No, now I'm definitely not going to give him a jab.'" He laughed cynically.

"Why was the morphine administered subcutaneously?"

"Because if we prescribe it intravenously then we have to administer it ourselves, whereas when it's subcutaneous we can leave it to the nurses." At this, he burst out laughing. "No, but seriously," he continued, when the outburst had subsided, "the nurses aren't allowed to give intravenous shots, at least not morphine. You administer it subcutaneous so that it can disperse evenly over a longer period of time. And we wouldn't have given it intravenously anyway because that would have killed him outright, and that would really be euthanasia. You would kill him outright; you know that it would kill him outright, and that has nothing to do with alleviating shortness of breath."

Martin Schuyt

"Yes, Mr. Oosten. I was only here during the first stage," Martin Schuyt said when I spoke to him later the same day. "I'd already been seeing him for about a year and a half or two years in my outpatients' clinic because of his serious emphysema. Emphysema without any malignity, a smoker's emphysema. He had really smoked a lot during his life. An intelligent man, who knew quite well what the cause of his illness was. As time went by, he became more and more incapacitated. He was already quite incapacitated when I saw him for the first time. It often happens like that, you know. Emphysema, elasticity of the lungs is gone, and when the elasticity is gone, there's not much you can do about it. It's progressive. His condition gradually deteriorated until he was hardly capable of doing anything for himself at home, and that's when he decided he'd had enough.

"So the last time he came to my outpatients' clinic with his daughter, he said, 'Now I've had enough.' I said, 'Now just listen here; you've never even been admitted to hospital'—because that's something he'd always refused. 'Who knows,' I said, 'if we admit you and give you treatment we can't provide to outpatients, and [if] we try some physiotherapy'—that's also something he'd always refused—'then we might be able to achieve some improvement. I'd like to try that before you even mention something like euthanasia.'

"So we admitted him. We gave him an infusion, and, well, it didn't make much difference. The man was convinced that euthanasia was the solution, and we just had to carry it out. And, well, I wasn't very happy about that because the man didn't even have a malignity. Of course he had a serious disease, but if you look at the population as a whole, then there are a lot of people with serious diseases like that. And different people can experience the same condition in very different ways. There are emphysema patients who can only sit in a chair, read, watch TV, or look out the window; they can't do anything else because they're connected to an oxygen cylinder which is too heavy to move, but they still seem to get years of fulfillment out of what's left of their lives. We have a lot of people like that in our practice. We discussed it with him and told him that we were opposed to euthanasia. One of his daughters who is a GP told us that the children supported their father's euthanasia request. I discussed it with her and told her that it wasn't possible at that moment, that we weren't ready, and that it needed to be discussed much more fully, especially with his GP, who had known him for much longer, and also with the rest of the family. What we did agree to—and we usually do that when their condition is that bad—is that we wouldn't transfer him to intensive care and we wouldn't put him on a respirator, never, obviously. And I also agreed, at his own urgent request, that if he were to contract something else, pneumonia, for example, then we would abstain from treating it. Then . . . then I went on vacation, and when I came back he was gone. I think he contracted pneumonia, and possibly became septic."

"That's another of those cases in which morphine and emphysema together led to death," I said.

"Look, in cases like that, it doesn't take much. . . . If you contract pneumonia, then it's fatal because you don't have any reserves. And if you become septic, which affects your blood pressure, then you become acutely very ill, and then it doesn't take much."

WHEN IS EUTHANASIA NEGOTIABLE?

Although neither of the pulmonologists was opposed to euthanasia, in principle, they were both opposed to it in the case of Mr. Oosten, for various reasons. One of the most important reasons was that Mr. Oosten was not in the terminal phase of his illness. When talking about the criteria for granting a euthanasia request, Dr. Schuyt made a clear distinction between emphysema and malignity. Mr. Oosten had a serious, fatal illness, but he could, theoretically, still survive for months in that condition. On the other hand, patients with advanced lung cancer usually only have a matter of weeks, or even days. (That is, by "terminal" they meant that the patient would certainly die within a matter of days.)

A second reason for not granting Mr. Oosten's request was that Dr. Schuyt did not think that his suffering was unbearable. Here, the question arises, "What is unbearable suffering, and when is the quality of life so poor that terminating a patient's life becomes an acceptable option?" For Martin Schuyt, the distinction was clear: Mr. Oosten was suffering and he would die within the foreseeable future, but a pulmonologist's practice sees a large number of patients in the same condition, immobile due to shortness of breath, dependent on oxygen from a cylinder to which they are doomed to remain connected for the rest of their lives. They all experience their suffering differently, however; while for some it is hopeless and unbearable, others still get enough pleasure from watching football on television or receiving visitors to make life worth living.

Of course, not every one likes watching television, and there are those who do not receive visitors, their loneliness and isolation being just as unbearable as their physical ailment. Suffering can also be subjective, and what counts as an acceptable quality of life varies from one individual to another. Dr. Schuyt was aware of these subjective factors, and it is clear from what he said that he did not reject them outright as a legitimate reason for granting a euthanasia request: when a patient has reached the point at which he or she considers the suffering to be unbearable, then euthanasia becomes negotiable, with certain conditions. The patient must have tried, or at least considered, the various options that are available for alleviating his or her suffering, or, rather, the doctor must be convinced that this has occurred to a sufficient extent. Dr. Schuyt was not convinced that Mr. Oosten had tried all the options available for reducing his suffering. He had always refused to be admitted to the hospital and had refused to try physiotherapy. Of course, it later became apparent that these measures did not reduce his suffering, but his refusal to try them suggested that his condition was good enough to be able to refuse possible relief.

These two points form the basis of much of the recent discussion about euthanasia in the Netherlands. During the past twenty years, Dutch doctors have been increasingly willing to make public how they assist patients to die. Dutch jurisprudence has developed accordingly, and although euthanasia was, and still is, illegal according to Article 293 of the penal code, a number of "rules of due care" have developed. If a doctor who performs euthanasia can prove that he or she conformed to these rules, then that doctor will not be prosecuted.

Although not explicitly mentioned in the various versions of the rules of due care, it was generally assumed, at the time of this study, that euthanasia was only justified in the case of physical illness (i.e., not in the case of patients with mental disorders such as depression), and if the patient was in the "terminal phase" of this illness (i.e., that he or she did not have very long to live anyway).

Changes to the law, passed by parliament in 1993, formalized these criteria, including the "terminal phase" criterion, while still leaving Article 293 intact as a safety device to enable the prosecution of those who neglected the rules. Politicians and jurists thought that they had now "finally brought the discussion about euthanasia in the Netherlands to an end." However, recent media attention has focused increasingly on a number of cases in which doctors have reported assisting in the suicide of patients with purely mental complaints who, moreover, had also refused to try various options for relieving their complaints. This reopened the discussion, focusing attention on the relative nature of "unbearable suffering" and leading to calls for changes to the new law.

Returning to Mr. Oosten, it is clear that patients can also give certain indications that support their claim that their suffering is unbearable and they no longer want to live. For example, patients may refuse further treatment or food. I have seen a number of patients persistently demanding euthanasia while complaining just as persistently that the nurses were late with their medicine and their meals. Family doctors told me that elderly patients often complain that they have nothing to live for and demand "a shot" so that they can die in peace. One doctor told me that, in response to such requests, he says, "All you have to do is leave the pills I've just prescribed on your bedside cupboard, and you won't be here tomorrow morning," or some such remark. Upon visiting them the next day, however, he finds that they have always taken their pills conscientiously. In other words, while some doctors may grant a request in the absence of terminal illness, a terminal illness together with a euthanasia request (even one that is persistent) is not sufficient grounds for a doctor to grant a request.

Later on, Mr. Oosten did ask the doctors not to treat any complications, but shortly after that, Dr. Schuyt went on vacation, so I do not know to what extent this might have influenced his position on Mr. Oosten's euthanasia request.

An additional factor in this case was that Dr. Schuyt was generally relatively reluctant when it came to euthanasia. He was open to euthanasia requests from his patients and quite willing to consider them seriously, but I always had the impression that he avoided it if he possibly could. At one point, Connie, one of the nurses, told me that Dr. Schuyt never visited Mr. Oosten. If this was true, then it was probably primarily because the specialists could not do very much for Mr. Oosten anyway. Palliative care was in the hands of Albert, the ward doctor, and the nursing staff, and Dr. Schuyt probably preferred to devote his time to patients for whom he could do something. Moreover, during the major part of Mr. Oosten's stay in the hospital, Dr. Schuyt was on vacation. Be that as it may, however, I do think that Mr. Oosten's persistent requests for euthanasia must have had at least some deterrent effect on the frequency of Dr. Schuyt's visits.

Mr. Oosten's announcement that he wanted the doctors to abstain from treating complications did make it easier for Dr. Schuyt. He could then abstain from active treatment, and the responsibility shifted to Mr. Oosten himself. (In the case of euthanasia, the patient decides that he or she wants to die, but the doctor is burdened with the difficult moral decisions: Is the request justified? Should the doctor acquiesce? How? When? However, if the patient refuses further treatment, which is the patient's legal *right* in the Netherlands, then the doctor *must* acquiesce, while at the same time being freed from much of the moral responsibility.) After he had instituted a policy of abstinence, Dr. Schuyt was obviously relieved. When he told me about it afterward he said, "I also agreed, at his own urgent request, that if he were to contract something else, pneumonia, for example, then we would abstain from treating it. Then . . . then I went on vacation," he gave a sigh of relief and laughed, "and when I came back he was gone."

Dr. Glas's attitude toward euthanasia was very different from Dr. Schuyt's. However, it is extremely difficult to describe and interpret these differences without using a terminology that also has other, unintended connotations. If I write "Dr. Glas was more open to euthanasia requests from his patients than Dr. Schuyt" then the term *open* suggests that Dr. Glas had a ready ear for his patients, that he empathized more with them. It might imply that Dr. Schuyt's relationship with his patients was characterized by the opposite value, *closed*. On the other hand, if I write "Dr. Schuyt was more careful than Dr. Glas when it came to granting requests for euthanasia" then the term *careful* might suggest that Dr. Glas was negligent with regard to the ethical, and perhaps even the medical, norms when euthanasia was involved.

Such connotations are completely groundless, but the loaded terms are, nonetheless, necessary to characterize each doctor's *style*. To a certain extent, Dr. Glas *was* more open to the euthanasia requests of his patients, and Dr. Schuyt *was* more careful. These differences in style were expressed in diverse ways. In the outpatient clinic, Dr. Glas regularly devoted hours to his patients, much to the frustration of the receptionists in the outpatients department. His morning surgery would extend imperceptibly into his afternoon surgery, and he would miss his lunch to let an elderly lady finish a lengthy exposition on her canaries. Dr. Schuyt, on the other hand, was capable of systematically limiting the time he spent with patients to ten minutes, and he usually finished his surgery on time. Dr. Glas visited his patients at home, outside working hours. As far as I know, Dr. Schuyt never did that.

Dr. Glas readily confronted patients' euthanasia requests and discussed them in a way that, I occasionally suspected, gave patients the impression, sometimes wrongly, that he intended to grant their request. This occasionally led to recriminations when it became clear that this was not the case (see Chapter 5). Dr. Schuyt always made it quite clear from the start that he was not keen on granting euthanasia requests and that the process was long and difficult. Dr. Glas's medical explanations were often extended, cheerful events, but they were couched in medical and intellectual terminology that, I thought, sometimes completely escaped patients, giving rise to misunderstandings. Dr. Schuyt's explanations were short, serious, and didactic, carefully adjusted to the patient's level of education and knowledge of his or her illness.

However, Dr. Glas did agree with Dr. Schuyt's refusal to grant Mr. Oosten's euthanasia request. He agreed that the patient was not yet in the terminal phase of his illness and that he was not (yet) suffering unbearably. Perhaps this was because Mr. Oosten was not his patient and he did not bear the responsibility for the decision anyway. It is difficult to speculate on whether he would have interpreted Mr. Oosten's request differently if Mr. Oosten had been his patient. I occasionally tried to explore this by drawing a comparison with the case of Mrs. Van Nelle, but Dr. Glas always insisted that the cases were very different in important respects, and, of course, they were.

Also, even if Dr. Glas had tended to view Mr. Oosten's request as legitimate, it is unlikely that he would have expressed it openly, as this would have obliged him to consider granting the request in Dr. Schuyt's absence, thus both contradicting Dr. Schuyt's policy (and thereby implying that his interpretation had been mistaken) and voluntarily immersing himself in a difficult situation full of ethical dilemmas.

Albert Meertens's interpretation of Mr. Oosten's request varied. When, after the weekly rounds on January 26, I said that I wondered why the specialists were ignoring Mr. Oosten's euthanasia request, he said that it also surprised him, that he thought that the case was clear, and that he would have granted the request if it were up to him. He did not think that it was all that obvious that Mr. Oosten was not suffering unbearably.

However, when I spoke to him later, after his leave and after he had given the order to the nursing staff to increase Mr. Oosten's morphine dose, he appeared to have a different view. Although he still thought that Mr. Oosten's euthanasia request should have been taken seriously (in the sense that it was well considered and not the result of senility), he now thought that Mr. Oosten's condition had been relatively acceptable when he had first requested euthanasia. (He could now compare this with his condition at the end when it had "really" deteriorated.) He argued that, as a doctor, you had to draw a line between what you considered to be acceptable and what you considered to be unacceptable for a patient, and that the criteria were ultimately subjective. He was no longer sure what he would have decided in the case of Mr. Oosten if he had had full responsibility. What is clear, however, is that the line gradually shifted as more of the responsibility for the actions that would contribute to Mr. Oosten's death was delegated to him. He became more cautious, and his position shifted closer to that of Dr. Schuyt.

As far as the nursing staff were concerned, the situation was clear: Mr. Oosten had a justified and consistent request, and the doctors should have granted it, or at least taken it seriously. This is clear from my discussion with Connie but is particularly striking in the nursing records, especially in the entries after January 11. Between January 11 and 28, the day that Mr. Oosten died, his euthanasia request was reported on an almost daily basis. These entries clearly show that the nurses were convinced that his request was justified and consistent. On January 14, for example, we read, "Really wants to die. Has only one wish, and that is euthanasia." The next day's notes read "Expressed the desire for euthanasia again this morning. Very clear!!!!!"

The nursing records also show that the nurses devoted a lot of effort to trying to arrange a discussion between Dr. Schuyt and Mr. Oosten about the latter's request. The tone of these entries is clearly irritated: "Try to arrange a meeting with Dr. Schuyt tomorrow morning about his euthanasia request. . . . Please evaluate euthanasia request. . . . Dr. Schuyt is still on vacation. Euthanasia request has still not been evaluated. He mentioned it again himself. . . . Evaluation of euthanasia discussion with Dr. Pool?"

Although Mr. Oosten *did* continually request euthanasia, the nursing records do seem to contain a somewhat one-sided interpretation. After all, if he wanted to die that badly, why did he not act himself? Why not refuse his meals, for example, or his medicine? His daughters also played an equivocal role, not mentioned in the records. One of them, herself a GP, insisted that her father's request be granted. But why, if she was so convinced that it was justified and necessary, did she not have him discharged and carry out the euthanasia herself at home?

EUTHANASIA AND ALLEVIATION

In the Dutch literature, a distinction is often made between ending a patient's life at his or her request *(levensbeëindiging op verzoek)*, which is still essentially illegal, according to Article 293 of the penal code, and death as a result of medication administered to alleviate pain and other symptoms, such as extreme difficulty in breathing *(pijn-en benauwdheidsbestrijding)*, which is considered to be "normal medical practice" *(normaal medisch handelen)*. In this context, it is possible, according to the health legal expert van Leenen, to distinguish between "normal alleviation of symptoms" and the administration of higher doses of morphine than are "necessary" (Leenen 1988:301-303).

The problem here is that it is not easy, in practice, to determine exactly how much morphine is "necessary." Pain cannot always be effectively alleviated (for example, when a tumor grows into bones or nerves); it cannot be objectively measured and is often not only physical. The fear of suffocating may be more unbearable than the difficulty in breathing itself. In practice, any sharp line between normal and excessive symptom alleviation is untenable. Moreover, discussions on the difference between symptom alleviation and euthanasia tend to ignore the fact that the necessity of symptom alleviation with potentially lethal doses of morphine *and* a request for euthanasia from the patient often occur simultaneously, as in the case of Mr. Oosten.

If these coincide, then the intention of the doctor becomes relevant for the distinction between euthanasia and normal medical practice. (There is much discussion in the literature on the distinction between primary and secondary intentions.) Did the doctor administer morphine to kill the patient because the patient had asked the doctor to, or did the doctor administer morphine primarily to relieve the patient's symptoms? The former would be a case of ending the patient's life at his or her request (i.e., euthanasia); the latter would just be normal medical practice. In the former case, the doctor would be basically acting illegally, whereas in the latter, the doctor would be flouting good medical practice and ethics if he or she did *not* administer morphine.

Intentions are, however, not easy to determine; they are complex and may vary from one situation to another, and an individual may hold different intentions simultaneously. Also, different participants may have different intentions. In the case of Mr. Oosten, for example, it is quite possible that Dr. Schuyt intended his treatment to be exclusively palliative, that Dr. Meertens was torn between alleviating symptoms and granting Mr. Oosten's euthanasia request, that Dr. Glas, when giving permission to administer morphine, also intended it as symptom alleviation, and that the nurse who actually administered it thought that they were finally granting Mr. Oosten's euthanasia request. As a result of this ambiguity, reference is often made to a "gray area" between euthanasia and symptom alleviation.

The death of Mr. Oosten also raises another related problem. When, in cases similar to his, the morphine dose is gradually increased so that the patient's consciousness imperceptibly dims into coma and eventually death, it is concluded that the morphine "contributed" to the patient's death, or that it "perhaps" hastened the patient's inevitable death. What happened to Mr. Oosten, however, was much more radical. When I asked Albert why they did not just give Mr. Oosten enough morphine to alleviate his impaired breathing, but without letting him die, he replied that that was impossible "because that shortness of breath is the very reason that he keeps on breathing. If you alleviate his shortness of breath, then he simply stops breathing altogether." His shortness of breath, was the stimulus that kept him breathing. Administering morphine to a patient in Mr. Oosten's condition is, then, tantamount to killing him.

One might wonder, in such cases, whether the intention of the doctor is important at all. After all, there would be no perceptible difference between the actions of a doctor opposed to euthanasia but professionally obligated to administer morphine to alleviate Mr. Oosten's suffering, and those of a doctor who decided to grant Mr. Oosten's euthanasia request, using his impaired breathing as a pretext for increasing the morphine. The difference would only be in the mental states of the doctors, and even this is an open question, given that it is unlikely that their respective mental states could, in reality, be neatly classified as being against or for euthanasia.

For Albert, the solution was quite simple: the death of Mr. Oosten was not euthanasia by definition: "If you decide to abstain from treating someone in his condition, and you only give them morphine to alleviate shortness of breath, then that isn't euthanasia because we don't call it euthanasia."

Finally, the case of Mr. Oosten suggests that euthanasia and the "gray area" separating it from normal medical practice may, in some respects at least, be constituted by the very introduction of the term *euthanasia;* that is in some cases, apparent ethical dilemmas are partly a result of our discourse. After all, this discussion of euthanasia and the gray area between ending a patient's life deliberately at his or her request and normal medical practice was made possible and relevant by the simple fact that Mr. Oosten had *requested* euthanasia. That is, the very fact of the patient asking for euthanasia made euthanasia a relevant issue.

We can go even further in this respect. That Mr. Oosten's death was *not* a case of euthanasia had more to do with how the participants talked about, or did not talk about, euthanasia (i.e., their discourse) than with their actions (i.e., what actually occurred). If no one had mentioned euthanasia, then the whole concept would have been totally irrelevant to the actions surrounding Mr. Oosten's death, but if everything had been exactly the same, except one of the doctors directly involved had described these actions as granting Mr. Oosten's euthanasia request, then it would have been a case of euthanasia.

Chapter 9

The Negotiation Process

PREROUNDS DISCUSSION ON THE AIDS WARD

I knocked on the door and, without waiting for a reply, opened it and stuck my head into the room. When he saw me, Dr. Edelman leaned back in his chair and blew a cloud of cigar smoke into the air. "Hans de Bruijne died during the weekend," he said. "It wasn't euthanasia, but Albert Alders, the GP, had to give him morphine." Dr. Edelman was sitting behind his desk. On the other side sat John de Wit, the junior doctor on the AIDS ward. Next to the desk was the trolley with the patients' files. It was Monday morning, and they had just commenced their preparations for the weekly rounds. Dr. Edelman pointed to a chair with his cigar, and I entered the room and sat down.

"I'll introduce you to Albert Alders when things have calmed down a bit," he said. "He knew the fellow well, and he's still very emotional. He phoned me at home on Sunday to discuss it. Albert always seems to have cases like that." He took a long draw on his cigar. "Bram Velser was also one of his patients," he continued. "He wasn't *that* bad, but he still came to me with a euthanasia request. I told him I wasn't prepared to do it. Goddamn it!" He looked at me accusingly. "It's a process that has to develop gradually. It's difficult for me as well, emotionally. I have to get used to the idea gradually. I can't grant every request for euthanasia, just like that. He was still in good condition, so I don't know why he didn't just do it himself, if he wanted to die so urgently. I offered to give him the means, but he refused. The GP eventually conceded.

"The problem with AIDS patients is that they're often depressive," he continued. "A lot of them have a history of psychiatric

157

problems. Take Frans Visser, for example. Just the other day, he mutilated himself theatrically with a knife. The doctor in attendance had to wrestle with him. And then there's our friend Bryan," he added with a sigh. "Before you know it, he'll be wanting euthanasia as well. But he'll have to try the anesthetists because I'm not going to do it."

BACKGROUND OF THE EUTHANASIA REQUEST

Bryan Mayflower had been seropositive for HIV since 1984. From 1986 onward, he had experienced a variety of serious illnesses. His case history read like a textbook of internal medicine: generalized swelling of the lymph nodes, oral candidiasis, recidivistic sinusitis, MAI *[Mycobacterium avium-intracellulare]* infection, PCP [*Pneumocystis carinii* pneumonia], Kaposi sarcoma's . . .

Bryan had been admitted to the Randstad Hospital on November 14, 1991. According to the case notes,

> Patient has had a 40°C fever for the last four weeks. Also headache, general malaise, weakness, generalized pain, tinnitus, diarrhea, dry cough. Now seems to have a recidivistic MAI infection.

"Appetite good," someone had added, optimistically.

On November 18, four days after being admitted, he mentioned euthanasia for the first time. He told one of the nurses that he wanted to discuss the possibility of euthanasia with the doctor the following day. He said he felt depressive.

During the following days, he spent more and more time worrying about his illness, and he informed the nurses that he wanted to see a psychiatrist. His partner visited him daily, and they went out walking. In the evening, on November 20, he left the hospital and went out to dinner in the city with friends. When he got back, he told the nurses that he had had a wonderful time. The following morning, however, he was miserable again, his body hurt, and he had headache. He also had an attack of diarrhea. Dr. Edelman decided on a different course of medication, and Bryan seemed to recover. He was discharged, much to his delight, on November 24 and was not heard from again until early April. His case notes of April 5, 1992, read as follows:

> Readmitted. Continuous high fever, generalized pain, headache, cough, sometimes nauseous. Severe diarrhea. Progressive abnormality in right lung. Skin irritation and itching, possibly an allergic reaction to medication. . . .

After receiving medication his temperature receded, and by evening he felt much better, though the diarrhea persisted, and he had to take large doses of Imodium to be able to reach the toilet safely. He continued to be troubled by headache. During the night of April 9, he started coughing up blood. The next day, a morphine pump was installed, and a week later, on the eighteenth, he was discharged.

On April 24, he was again admitted, this time to undergo a bronchoscopy. The next day, the nursing records read:

> Returned from the bronchoscopy at 11:00. Managed to drink something.
> Wants to go home as soon as possible (probably has Kaposi's [sarcoma] in his lungs). B has been told. Was shocked by this news. Feels that he is going to die soon.
> To have a lymph node biopsy tomorrow. Discharge Monday? Was angry and sad about everything.
> Feels very bad about his hair falling out. Today has just been too much for him.
> Wanted to sleep. Very tired.

On April 30, he was discharged once more.

Three days later, he phoned the hospital. He said he had a skin rash and his legs were edematous. He said he could not manage to get to the hospital that day but would come to the emergency room on May 7. He did not show up, however.

On May 13, he was admitted again. The rash and the edema had become much worse, and he now also had such serious backache that he had to use a wheelchair. He was coughing continually. This was the day that Dr. Edelman expressed his fear that Bryan might request euthanasia.

During the next prerounds discussion, on Thursday, May 16, Dr. Edelman took Bryan's file out of the trolley first. "Bryan," he said, and looked at John, with eyebrows raised questioningly.

"He had a lot of pain during the night," John said. "He kept shouting that he wanted to jump from the balcony to put an end to the pain, but that he couldn't get out of bed to get to the window. The locum was summoned but couldn't find any cause for the pain. He gave him morphine. This morning he raised the issue of euthanasia with me, but he added that he didn't want it just yet."

"I don't like that fellow," Dr. Edelman said with a frown.

"I feel sorry for him," John said.

"Yes, but I still don't like the way he forces you to do what he wants."

During the next discussion, on Monday, May 20, John informed Dr. Edelman that Bryan had now abandoned the idea of euthanasia. Instead he was going to decorate his room at home. Because he was now bedridden, he thought that if his bedroom was nice, then he would be able to cope better. Dr. Edelman was pleased that he seemed to be adopting a more positive attitude.

Nursing Records and Case Notes

Wednesday, May 22

Not very good night. Received morphine at 3:00 a.m.
Takes care of himself.
This afternoon much backache. Morphine at 15:30.
Was agitated (despondent) in the afternoon. Experienced pain. 10 mg of morphine administered at 20:00. Wants physiotherapy tomorrow.

Case Notes, Thursday, May 23

Results pathology lab: Kaposi's in biopsy.

Nursing Records, Thursday, May 23

Is restless and afraid. Emotional. Would like to discuss this with someone. John to arrange a consultation.
Has made arrangements for his funeral. Had a lot of visitors this afternoon.

Says his bedroom is going to be a "paradise." Says that when it's completed he'll be ready for what's to come.

[On Friday, May 24, John reported to Dr. Edelman that Bryan was now talking more frequently about euthanasia. If his Kaposi's was not cured within six to seven weeks, then he wanted euthanasia. It was decided that I should talk to him.]

Nursing Records, Friday, May 24

Had a good night. Dr. E. to discuss chemotherapy. M S Contin to remain at 4×20 till Monday, then evaluate. Robert P. is to discuss euthanasia, etc., with him.

Nursing Records, Saturday, May 25

Slept poorly, perspired a lot. Takes paracetamol regularly.
Feels great!!!!!! No pain, itching, etc.
Later: backache returned.

Nursing Records, Sunday, May 26

This morning, panicky and afraid. Wants to do everything and nothing. Said he felt lousy/down. Was emotional. Finds it difficult to accept physical deterioration. Wants to be able to do everything as before. Wants an acceptable life or euthanasia. Calmed down after talking to him. Realizes he can't make the decision yet.
No pain, thanks to M S Contin. Takes metoclopramide himself. Says he keeps feeling nauseous because of the coughing.
Evening: feels "mentally strong."

Nursing Records, Tuesday, May 28

PAC removed. Pain acceptable. Was tense. Received Valium. Buffy coat CMV [cytomegalovirus] positive. No treatment. Discharge tomorrow. To be picked up.

Nursing Records, Friday, May 31

Discharged.

Case Notes, Sunday, June 3 (Velma Veerman, Locum Tenens)

Readmitted via GP. Pain unbearable and couldn't be relieved at home in spite of increased M S Contin, morphine supps [supplements] and Thalamonal [Innovar].
Bryan says situation is hopeless. Requests active euthanasia when his brother returns from a trip (has June 15 in mind). Up until then he wants, after consultation with R. P. Edelman,

- adequate pain medication,
- medication to improve respiration, and
- all other medication to be stopped.

Temp. 38.9 oral, sick, painful, pale.
Conclusion:

- Unbearable pain in spine (low lumbar) in spite of extensive pain medication
- Kaposi's sarcoma right lung
- CMV viremia
- MAI

N B

1. The patient wants all medication that is not immediately necessary to be stopped.
2. The patient wants active euthanasia on Friday, June 15.

Policy:

- Continue all medication until Monday.
- Morphine 10 mg i.m. [intramuscular].
- Monday discussion about stopping medication and active euthanasia.

It was here that Bryan's euthanasia request was mentioned for the first time in the case notes (as opposed to the nursing records). It was also reported in the nursing report of the same day:

Bryan has repeatedly expressed the desire for euthanasia. He doesn't want to go on. It isn't just the pain, but having AIDS per se, and the fact of becoming increasingly dependent on others. He is to discuss this with the doctors tomorrow.

THE REQUEST

During the prerounds discussion on Monday, June 4, John reported that Bryan had been readmitted.

"He wants to stop all medication—"

"That's very wise of him," Dr. Edelman interrupted.

"—that isn't directly related to his back or his lungs. And then he wants . . . very much . . . to die on June 15." John mentioned the date rapidly, as though he thought that Dr. Edelman might not notice it.

"Inconvenient," snapped Dr. Edelman, and he looked, sulkily, out the window.

"Err," John hesitated and fell silent. "Actually, I think that the request is legitimate . . ." he resumed after a few seconds.

"Oh, the *request* is *absolutely* legitimate," said Dr. Edelman as he lit his cigar.

"His lab results show all kinds of abnormalities," John continued. He has hyponatremia, elevated amylase, elevated transaminase. I think that if we stop all his medication, a lot of these abnormalities will disappear. . . ."

"I agree, I agree," said Dr. Edelman, nodding. "But I also quite fancy the idea of giving him an epidural catheter, so that we can grant his wish to be free of pain."

"And then, of course, he also wants to discuss the . . . other matter with you today . . ."

"Yes, well, this doctor happens to be sick as well. He got up from his sick bed specially to make sure things were running smoothly here."

"Well," John said. "I'll stop the medication and ask the psychiatrist to talk to him. I've already discussed the epidural with him. So has his GP. But, you know, I wonder. . . . There's no substratum for his pain . . ."

"You mean you think the epidural might not help?"

"Yes, precisely. It's funny that his Hb [hemoglobin] keeps falling so rapidly. It's dropped again, from seven to five."

"I think the MAI is active," Dr. Edelman replied. "Is it interesting to investigate? Yes, from an academic point of view. Is it relevant for Bryan himself? No."

"He's got CMV viremia, he's got Kaposi's in his lungs and a manifestation elsewhere, and then there's the MAI. When you think of everything he's got, then he still looks in relatively good shape," John reflected.

"Yes, well, it just goes to show," Dr. Edelman said, "there are patients who seem to be doing fine and then suddenly drop dead, and there are patients who are really in very bad shape but who look great."

"But what are we going to do? After all, he does have that request, and it isn't going to go away. What's your opinion?"

"Look here. . . . The request per se is legitimate, but I don't like the conditions."

"You mean the date."

"Yes, the date. Something like that usually only happens after a lot of discussion. It has to develop. You have to get used to the idea. Only then do you start to discuss a date. Not the other way round. Not, 'Listen here, Edelman, I've made my plans for the fifteenth, so you'd better make sure that you're ready.' That's not developing together, that's extortion, something he's always been good at. So I think I'll . . . I'm not quite sure yet. . . . I'll think about it. Maybe I'll do it, or I might ask one of the anesthetists."

"Yes, I think—"

"He's been admitted again with the same complaint of pain. . . ."

"We've got the neurologist to have a look at him," John added, "but he couldn't find anything."

"During previous admittances, he would suddenly say, 'I must go home.' Then when he's been discharged, it's, 'I want to be admitted.' Always the same old story. He dictates when he's to be admitted and when he's to be discharged. . . ."

"And he decides on his own medication," John added.

"I've no problem with that," said Dr. Edelman. "We agreed long ago that he would have all that under his own control. But anyway, I must try and ignore it, that feeling that I get when I'm called out of bed in the middle of the night to be informed that Mr. Bryan May-flower wants to be readmitted and that he wants euthanasia on the fifteenth."

"Yes, I can understand that—" John attempted.

"But the request remains valid," Dr. Edelman interrupted.

"Yes, but as far as—"

"I'm not a psychiatrist, and that fellow needs help from a psychiatrist, someone who knows how to cope with such antics professionally."

"So you don't exclude the possibility that his request—"

"The request will be granted, whatever happens. When you look at his history, then he has every right to . . . his situation is unacceptable. . . . But sometimes I wonder. . . . If you're suffering so much pain, then how can you say, on the fourth, that you're prepared to hold on and suffer unbearable pain for another eleven days. I just don't understand."

"What I don't understand is—" John attempted once more.

"I don't understand it at all. If he said he couldn't take another minute of it, okay. The pain apparently doesn't interfere with his ability to plan and organize."

"I told his GP that there wasn't really any grounds to admit him this time, but given our past involvement in his case, I thought that we had a responsibility to—"

"And then the next question is, 'If it comes to euthanasia, are we to do it here or at home? And are we to carry it out, or do we let him do it himself?'" Dr. Edelman looked at me. "We could concoct a great potion, but there aren't many like Socrates who can actually do it themselves. I always give them the choice because I think they have the right to decide. . . . I can imagine that if you choose to die, you might want to carry it out yourself. I'll respect that choice, but I won't push it because I think that an intravenous drip is the best, both for the patient and for the relatives. It's finished in five minutes. It's a good death. Because you use curare, you sedate the respiratory system, and so you don't get that gasping that's so common in people who are dying and that's so horrific for everybody. You never get used to it: seeing someone lying there, gasping for breath, then nothing for what seems like ages, and then suddenly a gasp. It's horrible. Each time, the relatives think it's over, and then there's another terrible gasp. So I'll think about it."

"Do you think we need to do any more tests with regard to his backache?" John asked.

"No, given his prognosis . . ."

"Okay, I'll arrange for the epidural."

"Yes, and he's to manage it all himself. And just as he's allowed to take everything himself, he's also allowed to refuse everything. And that's the first step toward showing you're serious in your request. . . . "

Dr. Edelman's pager beeped and he picked up the phone.

John turned to me. "He always wanted the maximum dose of everything," he said. "And he always had suggestions for additional medication. So the fact that he has now spontaneously asked us to stop all medication is a clear sign."

Dr. Edelman put down the receiver. "Okay, enough of Bryan," he said.

BRYAN MAYFLOWER

After the discussion, John phoned the anesthetist, who agreed to come to place the epidural the same evening. He and Dr. Edelman then started their rounds. I followed. When we reached Bryan's room a couple of hours later, loud moaning could be heard from inside. Dr. Edelman frowned and said, "You go inside. I'll see him tomorrow when I'm less busy, then I can give him the time he needs."

John and I entered the room. Bryan was lying on his bed with his head and legs supported by large pillows. I estimated that he was in his late thirties. He was very pale and thin, though not emaciated, and had a broad mouth and large, pleading eyes, encircled by brown rings. His mother, a short, plump woman, was seated in the corner of the room, at the foot of the bed. John told them that the anesthetist would be coming in the evening to install the epidural. Bryan sighed and said he was glad that something was being done about his backache. John explained that it was not possible simply to carry out euthanasia, and that an official procedure had to be followed. He said that Dr. Edelman would come to see him the following day to discuss the matter. John asked him whether, in the meantime, he would be prepared to talk to me and the psychiatrist about his euthanasia request. Bryan nodded.

When John had finished, he turned and left the room. I was just about to follow him when Bryan suddenly sat up in bed. "Aren't you going to stay to discuss the euthanasia?" he asked. I had, in fact, intended to prepare some questions first, then come to see him the next morning, but his eyes pleaded.

"Okay," I said. "I'll be right back."

"You will come back, won't you?" he asked, leaning forward and looking me straight in the eye.

"It's so important for us," said his mother, as she came toward me and laid her hand on my arm. "I don't agree with euthanasia, but I don't want to see him suffer like this anymore," she said, in a trembling voice.

When I returned, I sat down on a stool at the foot of his bed.

"Come closer," Bryan said. "Otherwise, I can't hear you."

"He's going deaf," said his mother.

I asked them whether I could record the conversation. They said it was okay. As Bryan tried to sit up in bed, he emitted a cry of pain.

"He's moaning and groaning all the time," said his mother. "It's the backache. He's really in pain."

"I once decided," said Bryan, speaking very slowly, "that life wouldn't be worth living if I became bedridden. When I became bedridden, I reconsidered. I thought, 'If I decorate my bedroom and make it nice, then I might be able to hold out longer.' But then the pain increased, and they started talking about CMV and that sort of thing, and I thought, 'This is it. I don't want to go on. I don't want them poking around anymore. I don't want any more medication. I don't want anything.' I hope that John has already ordered them to stop all medication."

I told him that I had just seen John write new instructions for the nurses.

"So . . . so . . . what else is there to say?"

"When did you make that decision?" I asked. "Was it this week?"

"No, two or three weeks ago. I phoned my mother. 'Come quick,' I said, 'because I want to die.' It was an easy decision to make because of the pain and the suffering. I've suffered enough. I don't want any more poking around, no more needles. Except the one this evening. John says it will reduce the pain, so I can accept that. But nothing else. I'm finished. My mouth is dry from the medication. . . . Can you pass me that glass of water?"

I passed him a glass of water with a straw in it. "Did you ever contemplate euthanasia before that?" I asked.

"I've thought about it. Look here, I've got a euthanasia declaration that I signed last year." He leaned over and rummaged in the drawer of the bedside cupboard and passed me a document in a plastic cover. "I knew that the moment would come when the pain became unbearable. Actually, I made the decision about six months ago. Now I'm just waiting for the implementation. But I can't wait much longer because it's unbearable."

"Who have you discussed this with?"

"With John, my mother, my lover, my GP. They all agree with me. Now I still have to talk to the psychiatrist. I hope I can convince him."

"I don't think it's a question of convincing him," I said. "Everyone is convinced that your request is legitimate. But there is a procedure that has to be followed. You can't request something like euthanasia and expect it to be carried out the same day."

"I've already sent cards to my friends, to say good-bye, to tell them I love them, to tell them . . . to tell them that this life is finished for me." His voice trembled. "They'll understand. The pain occupies me so much it's driving me mad." He groaned loudly and looked at his mother. "Can you go and get a nurse to give me some more morphine?" And then, looking at me again, "Sorry for interrupting the discussion."

"Doesn't matter," I said.

"The pain is just unbelievable. But even before the backache began on Friday, I had already decided. Because I'm sick of taking forty-two pills every day, and having to lie on my back all the time. That's not life. I was always active. I did all kinds of things. . . ."

Bryan's mother came back.

"Is someone coming?"

"Gert is coming," she answered.

"The pain's driving me mad, not only in my back, but in my stomach as well. I'm suffering continuously. I used to be very active, so I don't want to live in bed. That's all I have to say. What else can I say?" He let his head sag onto his chest and was quiet for a few moments.

"I keep dropping off like that, but I can't sleep because of the pain. I close my eyes, but I don't sleep. It was like that on Friday night, Saturday night, last night. It's really unbelievable."

"Have you thought about how you want the euthanasia to be carried out?" I asked.

"I want it to take place here, through a morphine infusion. It would be ideal to do it at home, but that's impossible. It's better to do it here, then the doctors have everything under control."

"Have you ever considered doing it yourself? They could give you something to take yourself, for example?"

"That would also be fine. . . . But I think I prefer the infusion."

"Why is that?"

"Because. . . . it seems like a nice way to go. . . ." He paused to cry out in pain. "Goddamn it, what are they doing with that morphine? Mother, can you go and see what they're doing?"

When she had left, I said, "I think Dr. Edelman is coming to discuss your request with you tomorrow."

"Only tomorrow?"

"I think he wants to come when he has enough time to discuss things properly. . . ."

Bryan's mother came back, together with Gert, one of the nurses. He was carrying a syringe.

"In your stomach," he said.

"What?" Bryan exclaimed. "Why do you keep giving them in different places?"

"Maybe it's painful if they keep giving them in the same spot," his mother said.

Bryan pulled up his T-shirt. Gert slid the needle under Bryan's skin and slowly discharged the syringe's contents.

"Thanks a lot, Gert," Bryan said when he had finished. "I've just taken two M S Contin. John said I could."

"But don't take any more just yet," Gert said.

"I know," said Bryan. "I'm not planning to commit suicide, you know. I want euthanasia because my life insurance doesn't cover suicide, and I want to leave something for my mother and my lover."

After Gert had left and Bryan had coughed continuously for several minutes, he said, "I don't really have anything else to say, except that I can't wait for the day. . . ."

Shortly after, I left them.

On Wednesday, June 6, I went to see him again. The morphine pump was next to his bed, and he was in a cheerful mood. He said he was no longer in pain but was now constipated. He told me that the nurses had been giving him enemas all morning, but they were not having any effect. He was going to have an X ray later that morning, but he suspected that the morphine was the cause.

"How the hell do heroin junkies manage?" he asked. "They must be constipated all the time. Wouldn't that be a good topic for a dissertation?"

"Did Dr. Edelman come and see you yesterday?" I asked.

"No," he answered casually, as though he did not care. He started to talk about his life: his years at school, relationships, adventures in saunas and gay bars. He talked about his present partner. After several hours, the conversation turned to his euthanasia request. I told him that Dr. Edelman was not happy with his demand that it take place on June 15. He was shocked.

"I told John I would *prefer* to have it on the fifteenth," he said. "Dr. Edelman wasn't supposed to hear that. I didn't know John was going to tell him. I don't care when it takes place, though sooner is better than later. I only mentioned the fifteenth because that's when my brother gets back, and my mother wants him to be here. I would also like him to be here, then he can take care of her. But if Dr. Edelman would prefer to do it on another day, then that's all right with me."

"How do you feel about it now that you're no longer in pain?" I asked.

"Exactly the same. And the morphine also has its problems. I'm no longer in pain, but now I'm constipated. I haven't slept since Saturday because of my stomach, and I haven't eaten, only drunk water. I'm scared of getting even more constipated. And the prognosis is the same. I've got CMV. I can feel it in my back, and it's probably the cause of my stomach problem as well. I always loved music, but now I'm half deaf, and that's only going to get worse. I'll probably go blind as a result of CMV retinitis. I can't walk anymore because of the painful lymph nodes in my groin. I was always active, and now I'm bedridden. And whether the bed is in hospital or at home, what difference does that make? Life's not worth living anymore." He sighed loudly. "Actually, I'm ready to die. I've made all the arrangements for the good-bye party after the funeral. All I have to do is discuss the music with my brother." He fell silent.

"I know that the life I knew is finished. I liked to travel, but I'll never be able to go anywhere again. America, Portugal, . . . France. I'll never see them again. Have you ever been in Provence?"

I nodded.

"My God, Provence . . ." he sighed. "I hope heaven's like Provence, with all the lavender and thyme . . ." He fell silent and stared out the window.

"My mother's brother is religious," he said after a while. "Sends me letters saying that if I don't turn to Jesus, I'll go to hell. My sister sends me Bible texts. My mother also reads from the Bible and prays for me. In fact, my whole family is religious, except me. I do believe in the Big Tomato in the sky, you know, the one who pushes all the buttons, but I've never been really religious. I'm an Epicurean. I enjoy life, but the last time I really enjoyed myself, really did something I could do and liked doing, was at Christmas. I cooked a meal for my family. I like cooking. After dinner, I went to a few gay bars with friends. I smoked seven cigarettes and drank three cocktails. I hadn't done that for a long time. Now, I'll never be able to do that again."

THE REQUEST CONSIDERED

"And then there's Mr. Mayflower," John said the next morning during the prerounds discussion in Dr. Edelman's office.

"Yes, I still have to go and talk to him," said Dr. Edelman.

"I called the psychiatrist," John said, "but he's away until next week. And the psychologist wasn't available either."

"That's awkward. How's the pain?"

"His backache has now been replaced by stomachache. He's been given laxatives, but he keeps complaining about pain in the lower abdomen. It might be the morphine. We did a scan, but we couldn't really find anything."

"Amylase?"

"Elevated."

"How much?"

"It was . . . three hundred, four hundred." John paged through the file. That's why I wanted to wait until we'd stopped all medication, to see what happened to that value. But I haven't checked it yet, because he—"

"Doesn't want any more needles."

"Yes. I wonder how real the pain is. I often wondered about that when he complained of backache, which is now responding unexpectedly well to the morphine."

"Explain," Dr. Edelman commanded.

"There's no substratum for the pain—"

"I know that."

"So you wouldn't expect that administering morphine locally would stop the pain."

"We've done the stupidest thing we could have done," Dr. Edelman said. "We should have given him a placebo first. I mean, he said he felt pain, so as far as I'm concerned, he was in pain. Our problem is that we don't know what's causing it, and so it's important for our whole pain management strategy to find out whether it reacts to a placebo. So we could still give him a placebo through the pump, and then revert to morphine if the pain returns."

"Is it acceptable, ethically, to give someone a placebo to see whether it has an effect on pain?" John asked.

"My only argument is that one pain has been replaced by another," Dr. Edelman replied.

"Yes, given what he says . . ."

"How much noise is he making?"

"Varies. Yesterday I was summoned because he was writhing in pain, but I couldn't find anything. He didn't seem to be *really* in pain, just like with his back. When I went to check on him fifteen minutes later, he was singing cheerfully. So sometimes I just doubt . . ."

"It was on the basis of the pain that his euthanasia request developed, wasn't it?" Dr. Edelman asked.

"Yes, and our policy was to try and alleviate the pain and then see whether the request disappeared with the pain."

"I spoke to him yesterday," I said. "He was cheerful and not in pain. I asked him about his request, and he said that it was the general deterioration and the prognosis rather than the pain that were behind his request."

"That's what we wanted to hear," John said.

"Yes, that's clear," Dr. Edelman added. "But it's funny that it suddenly came up like that."

"He's had a euthanasia declaration for a year," I said.

"Well, so do I," Dr. Edelman said, as he clipped a lung X ray onto the light box. "If you're clever and you know what doctors can do to you, then you damn well make sure that you've arranged things beforehand." He and John contemplated the X ray for a few moments.

"That Kaposi's is not really improving, is it?" Dr. Edelman remarked.

"He's got three requests," John said. "He wants us to alleviate the pain, make sure he's not short of breath, and help him to die on the fifteenth."

"Well, we can reassure him on that count," Dr. Edelman said. "It seems like he's expressing a persistent and consistent request to both of you. So, I suppose I'd better have a few serious discussions with him then . . . Friday? The fifteenth is on a Friday, isn't it?"

"He only chose the Friday because he wanted his brother to be present," I said. "But he's not insisting on it."

"Yes, that's right," John added.

"He's flexible," I said.

"He doesn't want to give the impression that he's putting pressure on us," John said.

"There, you see?" said Dr. Edelman, with a satisfied expression. "I'm glad I decided to wait and give the fellow a few days. . . . Listen, his request is *absolutely* legitimate, and that's that. His prospects are nil."

"Yes, and by refusing all treatment and further diagnosis, he's made quite clear that he's serious," John added.

"Okay, then it's not really relevant to find out any more about the cause of the pain."

"So how do we proceed, with the euthanasia, I mean?" John asked.

"Ohhh . . ."

"What's the procedure?"

"Time-consuming."

"Isn't one of the anesthetists always involved?" John asked.

"No, not necessarily. The procedure I follow is that of the KNMG [the Royal Dutch Medical Association]. They have a protocol." Dr. Edelman rummaged through the piles of paper on his desk. "Here it is. Look, here's the list of things you have to check: Is the suffering unbearable? et cetera. But the most important thing is that you should make a note in the file of his first request."

"Done," John answered.

"And you must write something as well," he said to me. "Because it's important that he's said the same thing to different people. That's how we start. Then I'll have a talk with him, and if that goes okay, then we can plan a date that's convenient for both of us. Now, I've already checked in my diary, and Friday seems to be okay, but I'll do it in the early afternoon because I don't want to do it just before I go home. I could ask the anesthetist to do it, of course, but that would be cowardly. Because . . . well, God, I know I've complained about him, but he's not such a bad fellow, really. His request is legitimate, and as physician in charge of his treatment, I think I should take the responsibility. . . . And what's the other reason for doing it in the early afternoon? Because if you do it later, you'll be stuck here until late at night waiting for the coroner. That gives me Friday morning to make up my statement for the public prosecutor—I write everything down for him: why I've done it, what time, who was present, what I used, et cetera. That saves endless discussion. And then on the day itself, I also get the person making the request to sign a statement in the presence of one of the nurses. He also answers all the questions about unbearable suffering, et cetera; he signs, the nurse signs, I sign, and then afterward I give it to the coroner.

"And there must also be consultation. You're not a colleague," he said to me, "but you are involved, and that's why you have to write something. Because I make photocopies of all the relevant sections of the file and give them to the coroner as well. Then you have to find another physician who wasn't involved in treating him and get a second opinion. And that's a rotten job, I can tell you. I do it sometimes for colleagues, but it's not easy because you don't know the patient. Sometimes I also involve the psychiatrist or the psychologist, so I think I'll ask Marthe to speak to Bryan next week. I also ask the anesthetist to prepare something. It's usually a combination of Pavulon, Dormicum, and Pentothal. It's a good death, I can tell you. It's also a lot cleaner, emotionally, for the person carrying it out. But we've already discussed that.

"Then there's the relatives: whether they want to be present or not. I usually explain everything to the relatives as well."

"He told me he wants his mother, his brother, and his lover to be present," I said. "And that he wants it done through an infusion."

"What about informing the public prosecutor?" John asked. "Should you inform him—"

"Always."

"Beforehand?"

"Never beforehand. Because then you would be informing him that you are planning to break the law, and he'd have to intervene."

"And then something else. What if the moment arrives, and he says he doesn't want to go through with it?" John asked.

"Wait a minute. During the whole process of coaching you must emphasize that he can always change his mind. The request and the decision to grant it *are not binding.*" He emphasized each word separately. "You must emphasize that every time you discuss the request. It's never happened to me, I must admit, but with him, you never know. Okay, enough of Bryan."

PREPARATIONS

Thursday, June 7

Nursing Records

Discussion with Dr. E. and Robert P. arranged for 17:00.
Increasing pain in abdomen.

Case Notes, 16:00 (John de Wit)

In case of pain: increase pain medication via pump, even if this hastens death. Has been discussed with patient.

At 17:30, I accompanied Dr. Edelman to see Bryan. Dr. Edelman pulled up a chair and sat very close to Bryan at the top end of the bed. "Are you still serious about euthanasia?" he asked.

"Hundred percent," Bryan answered. "I also want to apologize for putting pressure on you regarding the date, but I've been suffering so much, I can't stand it anymore. I can't run and jump and play with dogs anymore, I can't cook for my friends anymore," he said, almost in tears.

"Listen," Dr. Edelman said, "I've come to make you a proposition. But first I have to make another point clear: that an agreement about euthanasia in no way obliges you to go ahead with it if you change your mind. At any point during the procedure you can call a halt without having to worry that you are embarrassing the doctor or causing unnecessary trouble. You can stop the procedure [at] any moment. Is that clear?"

Bryan nodded.

"Okay, the date—"

"The date isn't really important," Bryan interrupted.

Dr. Edelman cut him short, "I said I'd come to make you a proposition," he said. "When's your brother arriving?"

"On Tuesday."

"Wednesday and Thursday are out of the question. What about Friday, early afternoon?"

"That's great; that's just great. I'm so grateful to you, Doctor, for agreeing to help me in this."

"Now," Dr. Edelman went on, "there's a fast method and a slow method. Which do you prefer?"

"What's the time scale?"

"It could take ten minutes, or it could take half an hour. . . ."

"I'll take the ten minutes," Bryan interrupted. "The ten minutes are fine for me."

"Who do you want to be there?"

"My mother, my brother, and my lover."

Dr. Edelman asked whether Bryan had any more questions about the euthanasia process, but he did not. "But I do want to ask you something else," he said. "I've been having terrible pain in my belly, and the backache seems to be returning. Would it be possible to increase the pain medication to such an extent that I'd be completely free of pain for the last week?"

"Okay," Dr. Edelman said. "I'll increase it, and you can decide how much and when to apply it yourself. But I must warn you that if your pain becomes unbearable, we'll have to increase the pain medication to such a high dose that it might lead to your death. In that case, it won't be euthanasia but a consequence of treatment."

Bryan said he understood and that it didn't make any difference.

"And I'll be sending the psychiatrist and another specialist to talk to you. This isn't to find out whether you're insane, but I have to follow the rules of consulting colleagues who were not involved in your treatment. And remember," Dr. Edelman added, "Friday is not a fixed arrangement, but simply a proposal. If it was presented as a fixed date, then consulting them for their opinion would be unnecessary. Understand?"

Bryan nodded. "I understand, I understand."

"I'll talk to your partner and your mother later," he said, as he stood up to leave.

Dr. Edelman then went to inform the head nurse that he should increase the pain medication and put Bryan in control. "Then he can increase it as he sees fit, but you can also do it for him if he wants, even very high doses. And if this kills him—and I wouldn't be surprised if it did—then we'll treat it as a consequence of treatment and not as euthanasia."

He then asked me if I wanted to be present when he spoke to Bryan's mother and partner. I said that I did, and he agreed to inform me once he had made the arrangements.

Nursing Records, 20:00

Dr. E.'s orders:
Euthanasia next Friday, early afternoon.
Increase pain medication as and when necessary.

Friday, June 8, through Monday, June 11

Case Notes, Friday, June 8

Complaint right eye. Pain and burning sensation. Consult ophthalmologist.

Nursing Records, Friday, June 8

Abdominal pain. Backache unbearable. In consultation with John increased morphine via pump.
Really suffering from burning eyes.
Very satisfied with discussion he had with Edelman.

Nursing Records, Saturday, June 9

Slept reasonably well. Got up a few times to go to the toilet. Pain variable. Requested morphine to be increased to 2.9.
8:30 morphine increased to 3.
Washed and dressed himself.

Nursing Records, Sunday, June 10

Two considerable attacks of diarrhea. Sometimes doesn't feel it coming. Finds this extremely unpleasant. Doesn't want to spend his final days like this. Nodded off occasionally.
Asked for morphine to be altered to 2.5. Was drowsy. Wants to be more awake. Friend and mother visited. Bloody stools because of hemorrhoids. Sleeps a lot.
Eyes have been treated.
Trying to keep his spirits up.
Says he sometimes feels panicky. Loses control over himself. Says he's hallucinating but ascribes this to the morphine. Keeps changing the dose: now 2.4. In consultation with locum 2×10 mg Seresta [a sedative] extra, as a result of which he slept.
Continual abdominal pain. Friends sat up with him.

Nursing Records, Monday, June 11

Bryan passed away, suddenly. Phoned his mother at 5:30 and asked her to come because he didn't feel well. Was dead half an hour later.

THE MYSTERY

After reading the entry in the nursing report early on Monday morning, I made my way to Dr. Edelman's office. I knocked and went straight in. Dr. Edelman looked up. "He died suddenly this morning, goddamn it," he said.

"Yes," I said, "what do you make of it?"

"We had agreed to keep increasing the pain medication until he was free of pain, and we knew that there was a risk that he would die before the day of the euthanasia appointment. He knew that as well. I think it's better for everyone this way, especially for his family, emotionally, even though they weren't present. Euthanasia is always a heavy burden for the relatives. They often remain with doubts, even though they keep repeating that it was justified. There always remains a shred of doubt as to whether they've done the right thing. So, for Bryan, I'm glad it ended like this."

"What will you fill in on the death certificate?" I asked.

"Natural death. It was a natural death. Listen, it was a combination of factors, and the medication was one of those factors, but it was part of an appropriate treatment regimen. It would have been criminal to let him suffer pain unnecessarily."

"Do you also record the medication on the—"

"Not necessary."

The door opened and John came in. "We were just discussing the crazy events of the last few hours," Dr. Edelman said.

"Yes, it's incredible," John said. "I just phoned his GP, and he thought it was an appropriate way for him to go."

"Yes, just call his mother up and say, 'I'm not feeling well and . . .' And what it could have been, God only knows. I mean, it could. . . . Listen, the medication: not plausible. If you're so clear-headed that you can make a phone call, then it can't be intoxication caused by the medication."

"Maybe his lungs," John ventured. " The Kaposi's . . ."

"Or an embolism. Something like that: acute and massive. Or a massive infarction. Yes, why not an infarction? It's possible. In any case, it's a relief for everybody. . . . Last Friday, I was at my niece's wedding. It was two o'clock, and for a moment, my concentration slipped . . . and I looked outside at the beautiful trees and I thought,

'Next week this time, it's Bryan's turn. . . .' Well, he's kept us all busy, hasn't he? And then he goes and pops off like that." Dr. Edelman and John both laughed, relieved.

"Okay, life goes on," Dr. Edelman said.

Three days later, there was an autopsy. I asked John what it had shown. "Nothing," he said. "Well, not nothing. There was a lot, in fact, but no clear cause of death. . . . What *was* strange was that he was hypotensive. That could indicate a sudden increase in the morphine through the pump."

"On the Friday before he died, he questioned me quite closely about the consequences of him dying as a result of his increasing the morphine himself," I said. "He was worried that, if that happened, Edelman would register it as suicide on the death certificate and that his life insurance wouldn't pay. I told him that I didn't think that would be considered suicide. He was relieved."

DR. EDELMAN AND THE AIDS PATIENTS

Once all the arrangements for euthanasia have been made and a date has been agreed upon, it is not uncommon for the patient to die naturally as a result of the illness before the appointed date. This is not surprising, given that the actual setting of a date usually only occurs in the very final stages of the patient's illness (though the agreement to grant the request *when the time comes* might have been made months or even years before). So Bryan's death on June 11, just four days before the Friday on which Dr. Edelman had agreed to perform euthanasia, was not really unexpected, though there were doubts about the actual cause of death, doubts that were never really resolved.

Even though, much to John's and Dr. Edelman's relief, the negotiations and discussions surrounding Bryan's request did not actually result in euthanasia, they did reveal the details of the negotiation process as well as some of the social factors that influenced the process. I am referring, here, to various aspects of Dr. Edelman's character and some of the more general social characteristics of the AIDS patients as a group.

In spite of the hassle and the extra work, Dr. Edelman was adamant that euthanasia should be carried out openly and reported to the authorities. He had developed a routine based, he said, on the guidelines laid down by the Royal Dutch Medical Association. These guidelines emerge clearly from the preceding discussion of Bryan's euthanasia request:

- The patient must express a consistent and explicit desire for euthanasia to different people, and this must be clearly reported in the patient's file.
- The patient must be suffering unbearably, and his or her condition must be hopeless.
- Another physician who is not involved in the treatment must be consulted for a second opinion.
- The attending physician must discuss the request with the patient to confirm that the request is serious and well considered and to make clear that the patient can halt the procedure at any time. The physician must also make the practical arrangements in consultation with the patient.
- The whole process must be documented.
- After the patient has died, "euthanasia" and not "natural death" must be filled in on the death certificate, and the coroner must be informed.

Dr. Edelman's systematic approach was partly due to his belief that euthanasia should always be reported, to facilitate monitoring and control (and that this was necessary). In this, he differed from many of his colleagues, who thought that euthanasia was a private matter between doctor and patient.

Dr. Edelman's aproach, however, was also due to the type of patients he treated and the nature of their illness. Most of his patients were young and relatively educated, and they were well informed about their illness, prognosis, and treatment options. Indeed, patients were sometimes aware of new medication before the doctors. They had AIDS, and, in spite of the complicated differences in the development of each patient's illness, they all knew that the disease was fatal and incurable. The most they could hope for was to delay their inevitable death. Most of the AIDS patients with whom I was involved were aware of the possibility of euthanasia and of the steps that had to be taken. Many of the patients attending the AIDS outpatient clinic had euthanasia declarations, and euthanasia was a topic that was discussed openly.

One day I was in the doctors' office on the pulmonology ward when a young man in pajamas and dressing gown entered. He had heard that there was an anthropologist studying euthanasia and wanted to chat. He was well-built and looked fit. He told me that he had AIDS and, apart from a few barely visible patches of Kaposi's sarcoma, was relatively healthy. He said that he did not want to deteriorate physically and had already taken the necessary steps. He had read about euthanasia and decided that he wanted to have everything under control rather than be dependent on the doctors at the end. He had read up on which medications to combine to ensure an easy death and had traveled to Switzerland, where these drugs could be bought easily without a prescription. He kept them in the drawer at home as his insurance against unnecessary suffering. When he felt that he did not want to deteriorate any further, he would take them, and the threshold of what was unacceptable was low, he said. He was proud of his physique, and when the Kaposi's threatened to disfigure him, then that would be sufficient reason to act. He knew from the literature that the doctors would consider this insufficient grounds for granting a euthanasia request, and that is why he had made arrangements himself. A month after our chat, he committed suicide.

Once Dr. Edelman gave me the file containing the details of all the cases of euthanasia for which he had been responsible. There were ten of them—all young men with AIDS who had thought seriously about their situation and their prospects and had decided that they did not want to wait for the end. Their euthanasia requests had developed gradually, in interaction with Dr. Edelman, over a long period of time and during numerous hospital admittances. Hence, Dr. Edelman's statements about both doctor and patient needing to develop gradually toward the event together.

So, generally speaking, the AIDS patients in the hospital were well prepared as they approached their self-elected deaths. This was in stark contrast to many of the cancer and emphysema patients, who often had only a limited understanding of their illness and prognosis, either because they had not fully grasped what the doctors had told them or because they had repressed what they had heard. These differences were partly due to age: the cancer patients were a lot older, on average, and their generation had a different attitude toward illness, death, self-determination, and the expertise and authority of the doctors. However, a class difference was also present. Most of the AIDS patients were part of a cosmopolitan gay scene, and they came from all over the city, and even other parts of the country, whereas most of the cancer patients came from the working-class neighborhood in which the hospital was situated. While the average lung cancer patient read the Dutch equivalent of the tabloids and spent his or her days watching television or filling in crossword puzzles, the AIDS patients often had works of literature, art journals, or medical papers relating to AIDS on their bedside tables. AIDS patients read about their illness and about euthanasia, and they communicated with one another on these matters. They formed a *group*.

Many of the cancer and emphysema patients were not well informed about their illness or about euthanasia and related procedures. As a result, requests were often ambiguously expressed: "I don't want to go on like this"; "I don't want to suffer anymore"; "I want a jab." Sometimes they read something about euthanasia in the newspaper or heard about it from a friend and then requested it from the doctor, without being fully aware of what it entailed.

This is, of course, a generalization. Some older cancer patients were well informed (for example, Mrs. Kees, in Chapter 2, and Max Kraken, in Chapter 10), and some AIDS patients were not. The general tendency was clear, however, and the AIDS patients who consistently requested euthanasia had a lot in common. The result of this, together with Dr. Edelman's open and systematic approach, was that it was relatively easy, once Dr. Edelman had overcome his initial aversion, to set the procedure in motion and see it through to its conclusion.

However, given the characteristics of the patients, and within the context of this open and systematic procedure, euthanasia requests were, when they came, all the more compelling, and therefore emotionally exacting, for Dr. Edelman. On the pulmonology ward, the doctors could dismiss a euthanasia request as "not relevant" (Mr. Oosten, in Chapter 8). The euthanasia requests that reached Dr. Edelman were often the end product of a long process of reflection on the pros and cons, and discussion with friends and relatives. When Dr. Edelman's patients made a request, it was not easy to put them off: they were articulate and persistent (which was one of the reasons that Dr. Edelman thought that Bryan was demanding).

Dr. Edelman tried to avoid euthanasia, while simultaneously realizing that he could not avoid it. His apparently contradictory (and sometimes blunt) remarks about Bryan must be interpreted in this light: "I don't like that fellow"; "he'll have to try the anesthetists because I'm not going to do it" versus "he's not such a bad fellow, really"; "his request is absolutely legitimate"; and so forth. Dr. Edelman's ambiguous actions must also be interpreted in this light. He complained bitterly about Bryan setting a date that he said was inconvenient, only to suggest the same date himself later on, for example. When he did not show up to discuss Bryan's euthanasia request as agreed on the Wednesday, it might have been because he was too busy, but it was also part of a pattern. On a number of occasions, I heard the nurses complaining that Dr. Edelman did not show up for such appointments. One day, before I worked on his unit, I heard a group of nurses complaining bitterly in the passage about a patient and his family who had been waiting for an hour for Dr. Edelman to show up to discuss a euthanasia request. Velma Veerman's compelling remarks in the case notes on June 3 should be seen in this context.

WAS IT THE RIGHT DECISION?

Bryan Mayflower was "difficult." He demanded a lot of attention and was always complaining about pain, even though the doctors could find no clear cause. Once his backache had been alleviated through the epidural administration of morphine, it was replaced by abdominal pain. He complained about constipation, even though the nurses reported regular bowel movements and a scan revealed nothing. Nobody ever suggested that he was faking to get attention. "Pain is pain, and that's that," Dr. Edelman had said, emphasizing that the patient's experience of pain was central, whether or not there was clinical evidence of a cause. However, the failure to find an explanation for Bryan's pain and his rapidly alternating expressions of pain kept the flame of doubt alive.

Much doubt was also expressed concerning Bryan's mental stability, with frequent mentions of involving the psychiatrist or the psychologist, something that had not yet occurred because both were away. We can only speculate about the effect on the decision to grant Bryan's request of the psychiatrist's verdict, if that doctor had had a chance to speak to Bryan. The psychiatrist probably would have concluded that Bryan's mental condition was stable enough to justify considering his request well considered (that was certainly Dr. Edelman's, John's, and my own opinion), but it is also possible that the psychiatrist might have emphasized Bryan's changes of mood, calling the seriousness of the request into question. Indeed, it is not easy to avoid the impression that Bryan was emotionally fickle or even mentally labile. He went into town one evening and had a great time, only to be miserable and depressed the next morning. He complained to John about unbearable pain one minute and was singing cheerfully the next. When we compare the various reports, this impression is further accentuated:

- On May 23, Bryan was restless, afraid, and emotional.
- On May 24, John reported that he talked frequently about euthanasia and had given himself six to seven weeks to get over his Kaposi's; otherwise, he wanted to die.
- On May 25, the nursing report noted that he felt great.
- On the morning of May 26, he was panicky and afraid, but the same evening he felt mentally strong.

It is clear that Bryan's mood was fickle and that he had difficulty coping emotionally. However, his euthanasia request always remained constant. He was also consistent regarding the other issues relating to his death, such as his funeral arrangements, saying good-bye to his friends, and so on. Bryan did not *want* to die, but at the same time, he realized that it was unavoidable, and he was persistent in his desire not to suffer beyond June 15. He never expressed a single word of doubt about *that*.

Chapter 10

Unreported Euthanasia

UNCLE MAX'S STORY

"I've got a lovely caravan [trailer] at the seaside. I'd retired, signed off. I'd made my pile, and I'd had a wonderful year and a half with my wife. We went on [vacation], did what we liked. I'd always worked hard, been economical, so we had a good life together. Just the two of us. Kids all married, so no problem. But I was a heavy smoker and, I'll be honest with you, I liked to have a couple of drinks every evening.

"So, one day, I didn't feel well. There are days like that, aren't there, that you're a bit whingy [whiney]? So, then I got this terrible pain in my head, here on the right, just above the eyebrow. It was as though my right eye was being pushed out of my head. So I went to see the local doctor. He gave me medicine and said, 'If it doesn't help, come back the day after tomorrow.' So I phoned him and said, 'It hasn't helped a bit.' So he said, 'Come and see me immediately, and I'll give you something stronger.' So he examined me with one of those lights and said, 'You've probably got sinusitis.' So, stronger medicine. He said, 'If that doesn't help I'll refer you to an ENT [ear, nose and throat] specialist.'

"That was the beginning of June. The weather was miserable. So I said to my wife, 'You know what we'll do? We'll go home for a couple of days, then you can do the washing and that sort of thing, and then when the weather improves we'll go back to the caravan.'

"Then at home I got another attack of pain in my head. Pressure on the eye. It was terribly painful. So I went to my GP, Dr. Bruijn. I usually have a lung X ray every year, so I said, 'Why don't we do the lung X ray while were at it?' 'Mr. Kraken,' he said, 'you seem to be a bit short of breath as well, so I want to send you to a pulmonologist for a lung function.' So, okay, I got a referral, and I made an appointment with Dr. Schuyt here in the hospital. That was that. I had to come and see him mid-July. We went back to the caravan.

"Two days back at the seaside, I'm having a shave in the morning; I cough up some sputum. Blood! I was shocked. Maybe a burst capillary, my wife said. Then in the evening I coughed up more blood. So I kept an eye on things. Next day, shaving, brushing teeth, you know the routine. More blood. So I phoned the hospital. I said, 'I'm worried. Can't we bring the appointment forward?' Because there was more than a month to go. So they said I should come immediately, the next day.

"When I arrived, Schuyt said, 'We'll make an X ray of your lungs and do some blood tests.' So, when that'd all been done, he said, 'There's a shadow on your lung.' I said, 'When a doctor tells you there's a shadow on your lung X ray, then in ninety-five out of one-hundred cases, it's cancer.' He said, 'We'll have to confirm that scientifically first.' I said, 'You're right.' He said, 'We'll have to do a bronchoscopy.' I said, 'Then let's do it.'

"And so we did a bronchoscopy on the fifth floor. It wasn't that bad. As long as you do what they tell you. They spray an anesthetic in your throat and you don't feel a thing. So he was looking and rinsing and pumping and looking again, and I thought, 'Max, something's wrong; he's seen something.'

"On the twenty-eighth of June, I came back for the results. Schuyt said, 'Mr. Kraken, you have an incurable illness. You've got lung cancer, the small-cell variety.' I said, 'Sounds bad.' Because news like that is sobering. I said, 'What are my chances?' He said, 'Only medicine.' I said, 'What does that imply?' He said, 'Chemotherapy.' I said, 'Okay, so no radiation therapy, no operations?' He said, 'No, only chemotherapy.' He said, 'I've got a proposition. I want to admit you to hospital on the first of July.' I said, 'Is it *that* bad?'

"Is your tape recorder still running? Yes? Otherwise, I've been telling you all this for nothing."

I had broken eye contact for a moment to check my tape recorder, which was lying on the bed next to him. "Yes," I answered, as I took a new tape out of my bag. "It's still running, but the tape is almost finished."

Max Kraken was sitting up in bed, supported by large pillows. I was sitting next to the bed. He had just had the last in a course of five chemotherapy treatments, the effect of which was to be evaluated during the next few days. It was the middle of November, and I had known him since his first admittance to the pulmonology ward in July. This was our first formal session with the tape recorder. He had a powerful neck, prominent jaw, and alert eyes. He was completely bald. Loss of hair is one of the effects of chemotherapy. Some patients tried to hide this under hats, scarves, and wigs; others tried to make the best of the few remaining tufts of silky hair. Max had shaved everything off before the first chemotherapy session, and I had never seen him with hair.

During his first stay on the pulmonology ward, I had not spoken to him, only seen him talking to a doctor or flirting with a nurse. He was always cheerful, *too* cheerful, I sometimes thought. During rounds he wanted to know all the lab results, exactly which medication he was being given and why. He asked to see all the X rays and got the doctors to explain them to him. He had long discussions with the specialists about possible therapy, and through it all, he always remained optimistic. "Then let's go ahead and try it," he said, enthusiastically, every time a new possibility was mentioned. At first I suspected that these were expressions of denial, but later I realized that he just wanted life and was prepared to fight for it.

"Is it running again?" he asked when I had finally installed a new tape.

"It's running," I said.

"Okay," he continued. "So what did he say? 'I want to admit you on the first of July, Monday.' I said, 'Is it *that* bad, then?' I mean, I'm only a layman, what do I know about those things? 'No,' he said, 'but it's the holiday season, so we have space.' What else could I do but believe him?

"So I came to the hospital on the first, and for two weeks they did all kinds of tests. And they started the first session of chemotherapy. No problem. I could still walk up and down the passage forty times. My body was still strong. Second session: also completed with honors. Third session: suddenly a lot weaker. Now I could only walk up and down twelve times before I was tired and had to lie down.

"When I went home after the third session, I started to have diarrhea for the first time. They gave me a sort of magnesium powder, which made the stools dry. And what was the result of that? Hemorrhoids. And they were painful as well.

"In the meantime, I'd also been having radiation therapy because I'm participating in a scientific trial. I had the first two chemo sessions, then a week of rest, then a week of radiation, then another week of rest. Then came the third chemo session. Then came the diarrhea, which weakened me even further. Then came the fourth chemo session, and I couldn't walk up the corridor even once. I was too weak, get it? But I managed to complete everything. Never gave up. Persevered.

"Then came the fifth session. Monday went perfectly. Wednesday . . . I don't know what's wrong with the Wednesday. Mentally and physically, the Wednesday is always the most difficult day. So, next day, fever. Today, fever. So now we have to wait and see what's going to happen now.

"And then, of course, there's the mental pressure. You already have the physical burden, and then you get a mental burden on top of it. And then a lot depends on your marriage, relationship with the children. How are they coping? As long as nothing goes wrong, there are no problems, but as soon as the motor starts failing, then there's less understanding. Sometimes they don't want to—or can't—understand that you're sick. Get it?

"So, I've been married for thirty-seven years. She's a darling, but mentally not very robust. But we've had a wonderful life together. And now, suddenly, I'm falling away, and it's hard for her. If I phone home and she doesn't answer, then I get worried. I think 'What could have happened?' Yesterday evening I phoned three times. No answer. Then when she did answer, she was negative. I hung up. I was angry. Furious. I could've got dressed and gone straight home. But then I'd only make my condition worse. And who knows what the consequences of that would be. Perhaps getting angry like that was the cause of the fever. I was so angry, I was soaked in sweat. I'm not used to all this, you know. I have to cope with so many new things. Understand? Mentally, physically. I have to pull others, even though I've so much . . . I have to devote so much attention to myself as well. You can't cope with extra emotional stress as well. It becomes too much."

"Is it difficult to accept that you're dying?" I asked.

"I accept it. I *have* to accept it; I don't have a choice. I know I've got that illness. I hope I'll be able to extend what's left of my life by doing the chemo and the radiation, that the tumor, those cancer cells, will keep calm. But once they start spreading, then it's just a question of time. And that's difficult to accept. But when you're on a ward like this, that's all you see around you. You're forced to face the facts. You can cover your eyes, stick your head in the sand, but then you're being stupid. Because it doesn't help. You have to say, 'Make the best of every day.' Because the warning of *what* was to come was given on the twenty-eighth of June, but you don't know exactly *when* it will come. No one knows. But, remember, it'll be difficult for me when they come and say, 'It's metastasized.' Because that's the definitive announcement of the end. Do you understand? That would be the end of hope, the future gone."

"And that acceptance?" I asked. "When did you realize that? Was it at the start or was it a gradual development?"

"Right from the start. Right from the bronchoscopy. While he was still busy, I said to myself, 'Max, you've got lung cancer. You're going to have to fight to hold onto life a bit longer.' I went home—he still had to confirm it on the twenty-eighth, but I already knew; the twenty-eighth was just the official confirmation—and I called the family together. I told them everything. We discussed things, and I made my arrangements, right down to the smallest details. The mourning cards have already been addressed. Understand? Financial matters. Insurance, interest, et cetera: it's all been arranged. If I shut my eyes tomorrow, everybody would know exactly what to do. That's how I've arranged things. Listen, I manipulated things quite nicely. I managed to arrange very suitable health insurance coverage, for a minimum contribution."

"How do you see the future now?"

"That's a difficult question, a *very* difficult question. How do I see the future? There's a certain . . . how shall I put it . . . fear. Understand? Something every cancer patient has. The fear of the moment of truth, the moment you find out it's metastasized. Because you know that, sooner or later, it's going to happen, and you can't do anything about it. And that's terribly difficult, living with that fear. Understand? But I just have to live with it because I don't have a choice. But I do think about it. Listen, this brain is still functioning perfectly, and I don't repress thoughts like that. I think about it consciously, and that also gives me a certain peace of mind. So that's how I'm facing the future, that short, very short, and shaky future. It's not positive and it's not negative. . . . Understand?"

"Have you ever thought about euthanasia?"

"I've discussed it, right at the start, with Dr. Schuyt. He made a note in my file. I still have to discuss it with my GP. He's supposed to come and see me one of these days for that very purpose. The children will be present, and my wife. Dr. Schuyt made a note in the file. I told him, 'I don't want to look like one of those starving children in Africa, or someone from Buchenwald or Auschwitz, emaciated, and I don't want to suffer pain.' I've always hated pain. I don't like pain. Pain is unnatural. If you've got lung cancer, like me, which isn't painful, then there's no problem. But when you get to the end of the line, like some of the patients here on the ward, then things are different. When I'm like that, they have to give me injections so that I don't feel a thing. And when I'm no longer conscious, let them give me an overdose so that I can sleep for all eternity. I've no problem with that. I can't get better anyway. Why should they make me live three weeks longer when I don't even know I'm alive? There's no point. I've discussed all this with my wife and the rest of the family.

"But before they get around to doing that here in this hospital . . . they say, 'No, first an intravenous drip and a bit of this and a bit of that, and some nice tube feeding through your little nose.' And before you know it you're lying there, gasping like a fish. And what for, when you're going to die anyway? Why should they extend your suffering like that? Why, when you're going to die any minute anyway, and you've said your good-byes and everyone supports you and they don't want to see you suffer anymore?

"Mr. Benedict held out to the last," I said.

"Mr. Benedict held on to his last breath. But by then his body was completely wasted. There was nothing left of him. He was emaciated. His face was emaciated; his body was emaciated; he was cancerous from head to foot. Who knows the pain he suffered. I don't want that. I *really* don't want that. It's so senseless. Life is only worth living if you can enjoy it consciously, with family and friends, good food, nice cup of coffee, film on TV.

"I really can't imagine why the politicians are opposed to euthanasia. Who do they think they are? They're only where they are because we vote for them. They just sit there filling their pockets. They promise us the world, but as soon as they're elected and high and dry for the next four years, they suddenly turn one hundred eighty degrees. Listen, that's politics. Politics is the dirtiest thing in the world. Politicians liquidate; politicians enrich themselves. That's politics. It's the dirtiest profession. And *they* decide about life and death, about joy and sorrow.

"So, that's what I think about euthanasia. Listen, I know they're messing around with that euthanasia law, and that all kinds of scientists have to write reports. But it's as simple as can be. It's so simple. If you've thought about things, discussed them with your family and GP, you've written everything down, signed it, your family's signed it, your GP's signed it, then who's to prevent you having euthanasia? They say they're trying to protect you, they want you to hold out, but it's easy to talk when you're healthy. When you're the one in pain, you think differently. They should discuss that law with those who are really involved: cancer patients, MS [multiple sclerosis] patients, AIDS patients. *They* know what suffering is. They can decide.

"So I'm for euthanasia. Always have been, even before I was sick. If someone with a fine marriage, a happy life, falls sick, then you shouldn't force them to suffer. It's not natural. If you have to leave this world, why do it accompanied by pain? Why suffer?"

INCREASING THE MORPHINE

Max Kraken was discharged shortly after his final chemotherapy. A bronchoscopy in January showed no trace of tumor: he was in total remission. A few weeks later I phoned him at home.

"Robert here," I said. "I wondered how you were."

"Excellent. How are you?" In the background I heard his wife call. He called back, "Coming dear, it's Robert, remember, from the hospital." And then to me, "We're off to Utrecht today, to see our grandchildren."

He was making the most of the time that remained because he knew as well as anyone that the remission was only temporary. He had developed a good relationship with two junior doctors, Gerrit Knol and Mark Hansen, and during the summer, when he stayed in his caravan at the seaside, they had sometimes cycled out to visit him. They called him Uncle Max. Now they visited him regularly at home. It was in the context of these visits that euthanasia was discussed. They promised not to let him suffer unnecessarily.

One day in the early spring, I met Gerrit in the corridor. "Things are going badly with Uncle Max," he said. "Mark's been to see him at home. I spoke to him a couple of days ago. 'Listen,' I said, 'is it becoming too much?' He was already in pretty poor shape. He was hardly eating and drinking and looked tired and weak. He kept dropping off while I was talking to him. But he didn't want us to intervene actively yet. He didn't want to go to sleep yet. That's how he put it. I think you should phone him."

I hesitated the rest of the day. I wanted to phone him to find out how he was, to show him I cared, but I did not want him to think I was intruding on his final days with his family just because of my research.

The next morning, I overcame my hesitation and dialed his number. I expected his wife to answer the phone because he was too ill, or Max, himself, in the weak, drowsy voice of the dying. The phone rang. The receiver was picked up.

"Max Kraken," said a clear, cheerful voice.

"Max, it's Robert."

"Jesus! How are things?"

"Okay, and how are —"

"How's your research? Coming on okay?"

"Yes. How are you?"

"Excellent. They've installed a bed in the living room. I've got the phone next to the bed, and the TV. The weather's great, and I've got a view over the garden. What else can you want?"

"Gerrit said you weren't well."

"That tumor's growing rapidly again. But I haven't given up yet. I'll keep fighting as long as there's still some enjoyment in life. Don't you think? And if you need to interview me, come round anytime."

Two days later, Max became acutely short of breath and was brought to the emergency room. The doctor on duty wanted to admit him, but Max said that he wanted to die at home. He was taken home again.

That evening he was admitted after all. He said he couldn't cope at home. He could not eat or drink and was becoming panicky and scared. He wasn't in pain but was short of breath. Gerrit, who was on duty, said that he thought Max was afraid that he would not be able to take his pills anymore and that he would suffer pain. In the hospital, he managed to drink something. He said he felt safe in the hospital, in particular, regarding his agreement with Gerrit and Mark.

Later that evening Max complained about pain and shortness of breath. In consultation with Dr. Schuyt, Gerrit started giving him morphine. Max said that he still did not want Gerrit to "intervene actively." He was not yet ready to "sleep."

The next day, when Mark was on duty, there was reversal. "I can't go on," he told Mark. "I'm not going to make it. I don't want to go on. It's become too much. There's too much pain. I'm short of breath. I don't want to go on." Mark and Gerrit started to increase the morphine. Max became increasingly sleepy. His family waited at the bedside. As evening approached, Mark and Gerrit continued to gradually increase the morphine.

The following morning, his face had become gray and he was clammy. His respiration was superficial, and he looked dead. His pulse was almost indiscernible, and he did not react when spoken to. His family had been at the bedside for almost thirty-six hours. His wife sat tensely in the corner. It seemed as though she did not dare to look at him. A son had held his hand throughout the night. After a discussion with the relatives, Mark decided to give him Valium. He died a few hours later.

EUTHANASIA

Later I asked Gerrit why they had given him Valium.

"The same old story," he answered. "People develop resistance to morphine. And we'd decided that it shouldn't be allowed to go on too long. That wouldn't have been good for anybody. He'd also requested it emphatically: that if he wasn't able to make the decision himself, then we were to allow him to die humanely. We made him a promise, and we had to keep it. Just before he became too drowsy, he said, Remember, don't let me suffer, and don't drag things out unnecessarily.' And we didn't. We gave him Valium, after consulting his family."

"So it was euthanasia," I said.

"Yes, I suppose it was . . . yes . . . euthanasia . . . didn't report it though."

"You didn't report it? Why not?"

"Well . . . I suppose the fear of hassle . . . confrontation. And there wasn't much else we *could* do. He did have a euthanasia declaration and, well . . . I think it was euthanasia. You could also, I think, see it as a continuation of the palliative treatment he was already getting. But it does resemble euthanasia . . . active euthanasia. . . . But it's difficult to distinguish. He was so far gone, and we had the agreement not to prolong things, and the family was there. We discussed it with them. They were behind us, and they thanked us afterwards. But, according to the letter of the law, I think we would have had to say to the family that we would not increase the morphine any more once he was no longer in pain or short of breath. But that would have been emotionally and psychologically difficult for them. For his wife in particular. She was a nervous woman. You saw her yourself. She couldn't really cope at the end. She couldn't even look at him anymore. She couldn't say good-bye. She started to vomit and chain-smoked the whole time. I had to give her a sedative. It's difficult, when you see someone slipping away like that. . . . Uncle Max . . ." Gerrit sighed and leaned back in his chair. "He was an extraordinary person. . . . It might sound gruesome, but it's satisfying to be able to do something for somebody in a situation like that. . . ." A long silence followed. "Yes," he resumed, "in this job, you see a lot of nice people go."

WHERE WAS THE SPECIALIST?
DR. SCHUYT'S EXPLANATION

As with Mrs. Kees (see Chapter 2), the specialist in charge, this time the pulmonologist Dr. Schuyt, kept in the background and left the details of end-of-life decision making to the junior doctor. After Max Kraken's death, I interviewed Dr. Schuyt.

"Mr. Kraken had a small-cell lung carcinoma," Dr. Schuyt said, in his characteristic, didactical manner. "A limited disease, as we call it, which means that it was limited to half of the thorax. This means that even though you have a very poor prognosis, the situation is still relatively favorable. He received treatment as part of a trial, and there was a good response. He had a complete remission, as we call it. In January, nothing was visible when I did a broncoscopy.

"He then had prophylactic radiation therapy because when someone has a total remission, we know that there is a big chance that it will come back. The five-year survival rate is very low, and it frequently recidivates in the central nervous system. Even though you can't see anything, you give radiation therapy with the intention of tackling micrometastases, and that reduces the chance of brain metastases. So he had that as well, but, as it turned out, it only gave him a few more months.

"There was a reoccurrence of the tumor affecting the brachial plexus, near the shoulder, so the first thing he noticed was that his hand didn't function properly anymore—a neurological problem. The neurologist examined him and excluded the possibility that it was in the spine. It was painful. He was given painkillers and radiation therapy, also for the pain this time.

"And then . . . something exceptional happened because he. . . . He was very extrovert[ed] and had an extraordinary way of coping with his illness. He wanted to know *everything*, always. Right up to the end, he wanted to see all the X rays, even though what he saw was terrible. He had good contact with two of the junior doctors. They visited him in his caravan at the seaside. They took it upon themselves to tend to him in the final days. At first, he had planned to die at home, but when he decided to come to the hospital, they had a room ready for him on their ward. So Mark Hansen and Gerrit Knol basically took it from there. I kept in the background because they knew him well and because they wanted to do it.

"So what happened next? They did a pleural tap, which produced three liters of fluid, but that only brought a bit of relief. He became short of breath, and they started giving him morphine. There was no other way, really. It was completely . . . a gigantic reoccurrence— that's possible when it's small-cell. In a couple of days, you can develop a gigantic tumor load. That's what had happened. Yes, his remission didn't last long. It usually takes longer. You know yourself. There are some who can live normally for one or two or even three years after treatment."

THE REASON WHY

Gerrit clearly interpreted the death of Max Kraken as a case of euthanasia. If they had kept strictly to the rules, then they should have stopped increasing the morphine once they thought that he was no longer in pain or suffering serious shortness of breath. They continued to increase the morphine, however, because they had promised Max that they would do so, because the family knew about this promise, and because they did not think that Mrs. Kraken would be able to cope emotionally with a long drawn-out dying process.

However, the doctors could have increased the morphine as they did, thus consciously hastening Max's death, and still "kept to the rules" by simply reporting his death to the public prosecutor as a case of euthanasia rather than filling in death due to natural causes on the death certificate. They had, in fact, conformed to all the rules of due care and guidelines relating to euthanasia: the patient was suffering unbearably, was in the final stages of an incurable and terminal illness, had a consistent and well-documented request, and so forth. The only deviation from the rules came when they failed to report the death as euthanasia to the coroner. It is highly unlikely that they would have been prosecuted had they reported it. The reason for not reporting was the fear of hassle and confrontation, according to Gerrit.

There were also other reasons for events developing as they did. One was the personalities of the individuals involved and their relationships with one another. It was unusual for patients to socialize with doctors, and it was unusual for doctors to cycle to the seaside to visit patients in their holiday caravans. Max Kraken, however, was an extrovert, a sociable and easily likable man, and Mark Hansen and Gerrit Knol were easygoing young doctors who were receptive to informal social relationships with patients such as Max. Max was also sober and had clear ideas about what he wanted and what he did not want when the time came to die. Gerrit and Mark accepted and respected his desire for self-determination and, given their social relationship with the Kraken family, felt obliged to put this into practice.

Although Dr. Schuyt kept in the background, he was not opposed to increasing the morphine to hasten the death of a patient in the very final stages of cancer (as we have seen in the case of Mr. Strasser, in Chapter 4). However (as with Mr. Strasser), he probably would not have described this as euthanasia. As specialist in charge, this would probably have meant that he would have opposed reporting the death as euthanasia, even if Gerrit and Mark had wanted to, because he would not have interpreted it as euthanasia.

Chapter 11

The Social Context of Euthanasia

Those involved in the debate on euthanasia—politicians, legal experts, bioethicists, doctors, and researchers—often assume that that end-of-life decisions are made by individual doctors, regardless of the social context. This assumption stems from the fact that the discussion about euthanasia is so closely related to bioethical and legal issues. It is convenient to ascribe moral or legal responsibility for a decision (or rather for the outcome of a decision) to an individual. In the Netherlands, the euthanasia debate basically revolves around two questions: Under what circumstances is euthanasia ethically acceptable? How can it best be regulated?

I have shown that medical decisions at the end of life are not clearly defined actions carried out by individuals; rather, they are diffuse processes that cannot be precisely located in time and space. They occur in a continuous and indeterminate praxis: a "decision" (and usually it is a complex of multiple, often implicit decisions) can be seen as part of a "performance" in which various parties participate and in which verbal communication, different and sometimes contradictory discourses, and subtle and implicit interpretations play an important role. An adequate interpretation of euthanasia decisions is impossible without taking this whole "performance" into consideration.

In the previous chapters, I presented detailed descriptions of ten euthanasia requests and emphasized the unique and individual nature of each case. In this chapter, I bring these case studies together to discuss some of the more general issues that have emerged. This discussion draws on all thirty euthanasia requests that I studied during two years of participant observation in the hospital.

THE PATIENTS

David had AIDS. Once proud of his physique, his body and face were now disfigured by the purple-black blotches of Kaposi's sarcoma. Mrs. Kees had, at most, a couple of weeks left to live: with her stomach strangulated by a massive tumor, her final days would be dominated by continuous vomiting and pain, pain that could only be alleviated by the drugged numbness of large doses of morphine. Max Kraken was in the terminal stage of metastasized lung cancer, and although morphine had spared him from unbearable pain, he could see no reason for prolonging his final days when he was going to die anyway.

Patients who request euthanasia usually have a fatal and debilitating disease, and they perceive their situation as hopeless. Although there are notable exceptions (such as the much-publicized *Chabot* case—in which a psychiatrist assisted the suicide of a depressive patient who had no physical disease), most cases of euthanasia in the Netherlands involve patients with cancer, though AIDS and pulmonary diseases, such as emphysema and COPD, are also important. It is not so much pain, but a combination of fear, pain, and other forms of suffering; physical decline; loss of control; and hopelessness that lead to a request for euthanasia. Pain was the most important reason for requesting euthanasia in only 5 percent of the patients in a study of euthanasia in family practice (Van der Wal 1992:36-37; see also Melief 1991:55, 64-66).

However, not all patients react to physical decline, hopelessness, and pain with a request for euthanasia, and most people with terminal illnesses such as cancer die without ever mentioning euthanasia. So why does one patient request euthanasia while another patient in a similar situation does not?

These reasons can be found in the sometimes opaque and idiosyncratic personality of the patient, and in the vicissitude of his or her biography. The death of a partner, often as a result of a similar illness, was a recurrent factor in my research. Patients did not want to suffer as they had seen their partners suffer. Sometimes they did not want to go on alone after their partners had died.

The death of a partner played an important role in the euthanasia requests of three of the patients described in this book. David, the young AIDS patient, had seen his partner suffer and die of AIDS. He remained behind, alone, knowing the suffering that was in store and wanting to avoid it at all costs. Mrs. Kees had lost her husband to the same terrible illness she was dying of: cancer. Time and again, she reiterated that she did not want to suffer as he had suffered, and that since his death, five years previously, life had held no meaning for her. Loss also played an important role in the request of Mr. Oosten, the elderly man with terminal emphysema. In his case notes, a nurse had, written: "Wife died six months ago. Since then has nothing more to live for."

The fear of a lonely existence in a nursing home, the inevitable destination of many elderly people with incurable, chronic, and incapacitating diseases, also sometimes played a role in the case of older patients. This was an important factor in the euthanasia requests of both Mr. Oosten and Mrs. Van Nelle.

Other idiosyncratic factors can also influence a patient's euthanasia request. Mrs. Jonas, the middle-aged woman with metastasized colon cancer, longed for the escape from suffering that euthanasia promised but was restrained by religious doubt and the fear of offending the religious sensibilities of her children. Bryan Mayflower, the other young AIDS patient, insisted on euthanasia rather than assisted suicide because his life insurance policy did not cover suicide.

Patients' personal characteristics were also sometimes related to the type of illness they had. The AIDS patients I studied were generally younger; more highly educated; better informed about the nature, prognosis, and treatment possibilities of their illness; and more likely to want a say in that treatment than the average cancer patient. Once an AIDS patient had decided he wanted euthanasia, then he usually followed this through consistently. Much more variation occurred among the cancer patients: one day a patient might feel terrible and loudly demand euthanasia, but then feel better the next day and forget all about the request. Patients with cancer or emphysema often requested euthanasia in a crisis situation—when they were short of breath or in the middle of a "dip" during chemotherapy; for AIDS patients, the request was, more often, the final stage in a long process that started when they first heard they were HIV positive. Furthermore, the AIDS patients all *knew* that they were going to die.

Cancer patients, although they also knew that they were going to die (prognosis was never withheld from a patient), often still cherished the hope of a cure. Stories of spontaneous remission and hopeful but exaggerated expectations of results from chemotherapy, radiation treatment, or alternative diets sometimes played a role here. Also central to patients' euthanasia requests was the ideology of self-determination, which will be discussed later.

Once a patient has made a request, various other personal characteristics then influence the *reception* of that request, that is, the extent to which it is taken seriously and whether or not it is granted. Other studies have shown that patients with a request that is considered to be serious tend to have a more than average level of education, to have an active, independent attitude toward life, to be psychologically sound, and to have good relationships with family and friends (see Melief 1991). This is probably because patients with higher levels of education are more likely to share the cultural norms, expectations, social codes, and forms of communication with doctors, which makes it easier for them to convince the doctor that their request is serious. Moreover, patients with stable family relationships and many friends are more likely to give the impression of mental equilibrium than lonely eccentrics or patients whose relatives are divided on the issue of euthanasia. A euthanasia request from a patient without family or friends is also easier to ignore than one from a patient with many friends and relatives who can lobby and pressure doctors and nurses. The patients with successful euthanasia requests in my study also tended to be more verbally articulate.

These characteristics constitute a repertoire of social assets and communicative skills on which the patient draws in his or her attempt to convince the doctor and other care providers that the euthanasia request is justified. Patients lacking these assets are at a distinct disadvantage when it comes to negotiating their request, even though their claims may be equally justified from an ethical and medical perspective.

THE RELATIVES

In some situations in which the hastening of death was a potential issue, much emphasis was placed on the patient's right of self-determination, whereas in other similar situations the patient seemed to have relatively little say. Sometimes the patient's relatives played a central role in the decision-making process, but on other occasions, the wishes of the relatives were ignored. These differences were related to the patient's medical condition, his or her personality and that of the doctor, the nature of the patient's immediate social environment, and the type of life-shortening action involved.

Mrs. Jonas, for example, alternated between clarity and drowsiness as a result of the morphine she was receiving. She repeatedly told her husband and the nurses that she wanted to die, but she hesitated when confronted by Dr. Nieuwenhuis. Her husband and the nurses put pressure on the doctors to grant what they interpreted as her request to die, but the doctors insisted that they could only act on a direct request from the patient herself. If she did not ask them directly, then they were not even prepared to contemplate euthanasia, even though they believed Mr. Jonas when he said that his wife wanted to die.

In the case of Mr. Joost, the doctors seemed to act in the opposite way. Mrs. Joost said that she was opposed to euthanasia because her husband would not want it. This interpretation was tacitly adopted, without anyone asking Mr. Joost what he thought of the matter. Her demand that the doctors abstain if her husband contracted pneumonia was initially ignored, though they did eventually abstain from treating complications. She agreed tacitly with the gradual reduction of medicine, food, liquid, and, finally, oxygen. These decisions were taken by a collective of care providers, mostly doctors, in consultation with Mrs. Joost. The patient himself simply underwent these changes in policy.

Mr. Jonas wanted the doctors to hasten the death of his wife. The doctors refused, pointing to the patient's right of self-determination. In the case of Mr. Joost, everyone listened to his wife, and no one seemed to think of asking him what he wanted. Because of the nature of their illnesses, communication with both patients was difficult, but in the case of Mrs. Jonas, the doctors gave this as a reason for ignoring her husband's wishes, whereas in the case of Mr. Joost, this was the reason for negotiating (often implicitly) with his wife about abstaining.

The ideology of self-determination (see the next section) played a central role in both cases. In the case of Mrs. Jonas, the doctors made this explicit because Mr. Jonas demanded a different course of action to that preferred by the doctors, whereas it remained implicit in the case of Mr. Joost because the relatives wanted more or less the same as the doctors. Finally, and not insignificantly, the actions demanded by Mr. Jonas entailed active termination of life in the absence of a request by the patient (a punishable offense), whereas the actions that Mrs. Joost supported only entailed abstinence in the case of a hopeless prognosis (i.e., normal medical practice).

The doctors I studied did not generally allow themselves to be pressured into hastening the death of a patient without a clear and explicit request from the patient. On the contrary, doctors became intractable and reluctant to grant even a legitimate request from a patient once relatives started pressuring them to speed things up. Gerrit Knol and, later, Dr. Glas were reluctant to act in the case of Mrs. Lanser, partly because some of the relatives tried to pressure them to hasten her death ("You wouldn't allow even a dog to suffer like that," Mr. Lanser had said). Similarly, Albert Meertens was very explicit (although his remark was meant to be cynical) when he described the situation in which Mr. Oosten's sister asked him to give her brother "a jab," and he thought, "No, now I'm definitely *not* going to give him a jab."

Pressure from relatives seemed to have an effect mainly in cases in which the relatives were opposed to hastening the patient's death, the patient was unconscious or incapable of making his or her wishes known, and the doctors did not think that hastening the patient's death through abstinence was really necessary anyway. Pressure from relatives sometimes also had an effect in cases in which the patient was conscious and capable of making his of her wishes known and wanted euthanasia, while the relatives were opposed. The argument here was that the patient would die soon anyway, but the relatives would remain behind with the emotional consequences. In such cases, the relatives' opposition was utilized to support a decision not to grant the patient's request.

This is a very different picture from the one often drawn in American literature on end-of-life decisions. Jacquelyn Slomka, for example, writes, "Although shared decision making and patient autonomy are said to be important considerations in ethical decision making, it is often the family's wishes, rather than the patient's, that will be honored" (1992:253). Discussion with the patient is thus replaced by discussion with the relatives, and, in this way, the doctor complies symbolically with his or her moral and legal obligation to discuss prognosis and treatment with the patient. Although this might sometimes apply to patients in intensive care in the Netherlands, as was the case to some extent with Mr. Joost, Slomka's conclusion that "the negotiation of death is, in most cases, a negotiation between physician and family" (Ibid.) is totally alien to the Dutch situation.

In the American literature, the expression "the family remains behind when the patient is dead" has a completely different meaning. It is an expression of concern by the doctor that the relatives might institute a lawsuit once the patient is dead. The obsession with lawsuits and the role that the fear of lawsuits plays in medical decisions at the end of life are also totally inapplicable to the Dutch situation (although the fear of prosecution did influence doctors' willingness to report cases of euthanasia).

THE IDEOLOGY OF EASY DEATH

"I don't want to look like one of those starving children in Africa," Max Kraken said, "or someone from Buchenwald or Auschwitz, emaciated, and I don't want to suffer pain. I've always hated pain. I don't like pain. Pain is unnatural. . . . Why should they make me live three weeks longer when I don't even know I'm alive? There's no point." In Bryan Mayflower's case notes, someone had written, "Finds it difficult to accept physical deterioration. Wants to be able to do everything as before. Wants an acceptable life or euthanasia."

The euthanasia requests that I studied developed against the background of what I will call an ideology of easy death. According to this ideology, all forms of suffering, pain, and physical and mental decline have become unacceptable. If the means of avoiding them are available, why suffer unnecessarily, when you are going to die shortly anyway? This is a secular, hedonistic ideology that has banished pain and suffering and makes no attempt to search for some higher purpose behind the suffering. Although, in practice, patients usually shifted the boundary of what counted as an acceptable level of suffering and physical decline as their illness progressed, many eventually reached a point at which they felt that the crucial limit had been reached, that the small pleasures which they might still enjoy for the short time that remained no longer justified any further suffering.

During my research, I only ever spoke to one patient, a young man with AIDS, who wanted to follow the natural trajectory of his illness and consciously experience the process leading up to his death (though even he had the condition that this must not involve too much suffering, and he had a euthanasia arrangement with his GP just in case). Even people who had thought deeply about life and death and the meaning of suffering often came to the conclusion that suffering served no useful purpose, and that, even in the absence of significant suffering, when faced with an incurable disease, it was better to die at a moment of your own choosing than to slowly deteriorate while passively awaiting the inevitable end.

Patients sometimes believed that they had a *right* to die and that doctors had a concomitant *obligation* to assist them. This belief sheds light on why patients in this study were sometimes so adamant in their demand for euthanasia and so little inclined to reflect on what this meant, emotionally, for the doctor carrying it out. Patients who requested euthanasia sometimes hardly knew what euthanasia was (i.e., they were unaware of the rather narrow definition used in the Dutch euthanasia debate and the various rules and regulations, and of the procedures that had to be followed). Many had heard about euthanasia only briefly, in television programs, or had read the odd article in the newspaper, the details now largely forgotten. For some patients, the national euthanasia debate and all the media coverage seemed to suggest that patients with incurable illness, particularly cancer, were *supposed* to ask for euthanasia.

Superficial contact with the Dutch Association for Voluntary Euthanasia seemed to stimulate this perception. There were patients who, after hearing something superficial about euthanasia in the media, joined the association and signed a euthanasia declaration, without really understanding what this involved. (Perhaps they had been adequately counseled by the association but had forgotten the details by the time they were actually diagnosed as terminally ill.)

For example, when one patient (not one of the case studies presented in this book) suffered a bad "dip" during chemotherapy, he immediately started yelling that he wanted euthanasia. "I'm a member of the association [the Association for Voluntary Euthanasia]," he shouted. "I'm going to phone them, and they'll come and give me a jab. I've got a euthanasia declaration; that's what I signed up for." I had the impression that he thought he had signed a sort of contract that guaranteed him euthanasia as soon as he requested it, that all he had to do was call the association, show his signed declaration, and someone would come along with a large syringe to deliver him from his suffering.

The ideology of easy death was also evident in the attitude of some relatives. I sometimes heard relatives of dying patients exclaim impatiently, "How long does this have to last, Doctor? Can't you speed it up a bit?" and "You wouldn't let a dog suffer like that; you'd give it a jab." This was more often expressed in altruistic terms: "Can you give him a jab. I don't want him to suffer any longer." Sometimes this was true, but I often had the impression that it was the healthy relatives who didn't want to suffer anymore: they could no longer take the emotional strain, even after a relatively short illness. It was striking how easily some relatives reached their emotional limits and saw an easy death, "a jab," as *the* solution.

The ideology of easy death also leaves little room for spiritual counselors, and this might be the reason why they are absent from the case studies presented in previous chapters. I am not claiming that there is no room for spiritual reflection in a secular urban context, or that patients in the hospital never discussed their problems with spiritual counselors. Indeed, I often passed the pastor, the priest, and that strange product of the Dutch desire for secular reflection on the meaning of life, the humanistic counselor, on their way to or from a rendezvous with some terminally ill patient. However, it remains striking that I never encountered them in the process of end-of-life decision making, and that terminal patients hardly ever spoke of them to me, though they did frequently mention the hospital psychologist.

CONTROL AND THE NEGOTIATION
OF A GOOD DEATH

When I asked David whether he was afraid to die, he said, "No, but the way in which I die scares me. But once you know that you can decide yourself. . . . That's the important thing. . . . " Later, when I stopped in to see him, just after he and Dr. Edelman had agreed on a date for euthanasia, he said, "I'm glad that everything has been arranged and I can relax now. It's a relief to know that it's all settled and that I have the certainty." Certainty about the time and manner of death and the knowledge that you can determine this yourself were central themes in almost all the euthanasia requests I studied.

This is perhaps the most extreme expression of a key aspect of Dutch culture: the desire to have things under one's own control, formalized in the "right to self-determination" and frequently expressed in everyday discourse as "I'll arrange that myself" (dat regel ik zelf wel). Ignorance of this is at the root of the Anglo-American failure to understand Dutch euthanasia. One of the major criticisms of euthanasia in the Netherlands, exemplified in criticism of the documentary film Death on Request, is that euthanasia requests stem from poor pain medication and inadequate terminal care, and that if a patient who requests euthanasia, such as the ALS patient in the film, could be transferred to a British hospice, for example, the desire for euthanasia would disappear.

This misses the point completely. Not all patients who request euthanasia are in pain and without adequate psychological support; they simply want to choose the moment of death themselves. The patient in the film was not suffering unbearable pain, but he knew he was going to die and wanted to do so on his birthday, in the evening, after having a glass of Genever (Dutch gin) with his wife and doctor. Although patients in my study often spoke of not wanting to suffer pain, in practice, some chose to suffer pain rather than be pain free but drowsy from the morphine.

Euthanasia requests and related planning often long preceded actual physical decline. Although most patients with incurable, life-threatening diseases, such as cancer, never mentioned euthanasia at all, those who did broach the subject often did so at the very beginning of their illness trajectory, as soon as it became clear that they were incurably ill. These are "long-term" euthanasia requests, and when the doctor agrees that euthanasia is negotiable and would be considered, if the patient so desired, they are seen as a kind of insurance against unnecessary suffering and physical decline. The negotiation of such long-term agreements is motivated by the desire to "have things under control."

The anthropological and sociological literature on death and dying includes much discussion of good and bad deaths. Although the meanings of these terms vary from one culture to another, the different versions of good and bad deaths do have a core of shared meaning.

Probably the most extensive discussion of good and bad deaths is to be found in the anthropological literature. Here, lack of control and unpredictability are often the most important aspects of bad death (see Bloch and Parry 1982:15). All kinds of violent and unexpected death may be referred to as bad death. Bad death is unexpected death for which the deceased has not been able to prepare himself or herself (Parry 1982:83). Bad deaths occur "outside," away from family and loved ones (Middleton 1982:143).

Bad death is often opposed to good or natural death in which, after a full life, a person comes to a peaceful and predictable end surrounded by family and friends. In Hinduism, according to Parry, the good death is one to which the individual voluntarily submits himself or herself (1982:82). A good death is one that occurs at the right time and in the proper setting. For example, among the Ugandan Lugbara, a good death is when a man dies at the time that he has foreseen so that his sons and brothers can be present (Middleton 1982:142).

In the sociological literature on death, the notion of good death tends to overshadow that of bad death. Kellehear, for example, defines good death as "a set of culturally sanctioned and prescribed behaviors set in motion by the dying and designed to make death meaningful for as many concerned as possible" (Kellehear 1990:29). In this definition, the crucial element is that the dying themselves "set the tone" for their own deaths.

In the Dutch context, death as a result of a long, wasting disease over which the sufferer has no control shares many of the characteristics of bad death in non-Western cultures, and euthanasia, increasingly, is coming to be seen as offering an alternative good death.

Control over one's death is *the* defining characteristic of good death, but, somewhat paradoxically, suicide, though it gives total control, also increases the risk of suffering: a botched suicide attempt could cause increased physical suffering and humiliation for the individual and emotional stress for relatives and friends, and it may cause physical damage that will increase the very dependence and lack of control that were the reason for the attempt in the first place. To avoid such risks, the individual sacrifices (the possibility of) total control to (partial) dependence on the medical system, with the concomitant guarantee of painless release.

This release, however, does not come as a matter of course: it has to be actively and persistently negotiated, with the patient taking the initiative and the moral responsibility for the choice.

THE DOCTORS

When it became apparent that it would be difficult to arrange home care for Mrs. Van Nelle, and after a discussion with her in which she complained about pain, Dr. Glas decided to transfer her to his ward so that he could "really alleviate her pain." This alleviation entailed an increase in the morphine she was receiving that would be enough to make her "fall asleep" (*inslapen,* which in Dutch also means "to die," which was what she had been demanding all along). When she seemed to hesitate, Dr. Glas did not contemplate abandoning the whole exercise but simply waited until she herself indicated that she was now ready for the morphine to be increased. Once she was asleep and (we must assume) no longer in pain, Dr. Glas continued to increase the morphine, and Mrs. Van Nelle died.

Mrs. Van Nelle's case was complex, but after her death, the other doctors, many of the nurses, and Mr. Van Nelle all agreed that Dr. Glas had acted correctly, that he had done what Mrs. Van Nelle wanted. I also had the feeling that I understood why Dr. Glas had acted in the way he did. Later, in the case of Mrs. Lanser, I tried to anticipate what Dr. Glas would do. Mrs. Lanser seemed to be in a similar situation to Mrs. Van Nelle: she had terminal emphysema, was short of breath, and wanted to die. Dr. Glas seemed to be receptive. "I understand your wish, and I support you completely," he told her when she said she wanted to die. "Your body is worn out, and we can't do anything more to help you. This suffering has become hopeless." Later he told her relatives, "There's no need to drag things out. I'll give instructions to stop all medication, except what is necessary for symptom alleviation, and I'll increase the oxygen. That will cause her to drop peacefully into a CO_2 narcosis." This is the same kind of language that Dr. Glas used with Mrs. Van Nelle, but in the case of Mrs. Lanser, he did not follow through.

Why did Dr. Glas continue increasing the morphine in the case of Mrs. Van Nelle when no one else would take that responsibility? And why did he hesitate in the case of Mrs. Lanser, in spite of the fact that she was terminally ill and had a clear and consistent euthanasia request? The conditions under which and the reasons why a doctor agrees to comply with a patient's euthanasia request are complex and often difficult to fathom. The patient's medical condition and prognosis, the nature of his or her request, his or her social environment and personality, the personality and attitudes of the doctor, the nature of the doctor-patient relationship, previous experience with euthanasia, the attitude of colleagues and nurses, the specific subculture of the hospital and the ward, rules and regulations relating to euthanasia (and how the doctor interprets them)— all play a role.

I asked Dr. Glas why he was more reserved in the case of Mrs. Lanser than he was with Mrs. Van Nelle. "The family," he answered, after a long silence. And then, after another few minutes, "Mrs. Van Nelle was a *very* different case. She was fully conscious, she was in pain, and suffering unbearably. With Mrs. Lanser it's different. She's asleep and doesn't feel a thing. . . . There isn't a set of rules for cases like that; you have to judge each one separately."

This answer was not entirely satisfactory because after Mrs. Van Nelle had fallen into a deep sleep, and apparently did not feel anything either, Dr. Glas continued to increase the morphine until she died. In the case of Mrs. Lanser, the misunderstanding between Dr. Glas and the locum tenens about increasing the morphine undoubtedly played a role, as did the doubts of some of her relatives. But was that all? Some of the nurses also thought that Dr. Glas had been relatively hesitant in the case of Mrs. Lanser. One of them even suggested that this was some kind of compensation for having acted so decisively in the case of Mrs. Van Nelle.

In spite of my attempts to get a "total picture," what I experienced of the lives and suffering of people such as Mrs. Van Nelle remained limited. Mrs. Van Nelle and Mrs. Lanser had both been attending Dr. Glas's outpatient clinic for years. He had visited them at home often, knew their families well, and had discussed questions of life and death with them exhaustively. I had a broad perspective, I spoke to all those involved, and I could observe Dr. Glas and place his actions in a wider context. In other respects, however, my perspective was relatively limited. Dr. Glas knew his patients so well that perhaps he was able to observe and interpret subtle shifts of opinion and hidden strains in the relationships within the family and translate these into actions and changes in policy that remained opaque to a relative outsider. Perhaps he had been incapable of making these reasons adequately explicit to me, or perhaps he was not fully aware of them himself.

Gerrit Knol, the junior doctor on the pulmonology ward, also reacted differently to what I had anticipated in the case of Mrs. Lanser. This was just after the death of Mr. Strasser, in which Gerrit had played an active role. Mr. Strasser's reaction to his terminal illness had been denial, almost right up to the very last day. When Gerrit arrived on the pulmonology ward after his vacation, he immediately started to sound out Mr. Strasser regarding his attitude toward his prognosis. As I have already stressed in my discussion of that case, it would be going too far to suggest that Gerrit was provoking a request for euthanasia, but he was certainly giving Mr. Strasser plenty of room to express such a request, should he feel so inclined. When Mr. Strasser said that he had had enough and did not want to suffer any longer, Gerrit immediately interpreted this as a euthanasia request.

I personally thought that Mrs. Lanser's request was a lot clearer than Mr. Strasser's, but in her case, Gerrit was hesitant right from the start. When Mrs. Lanser requested euthanasia and the nurses demanded that something be done, Gerrit told them that he could not make any decisions and that they would have to wait for Dr. Glas. When I asked him why he had reacted so differently in the two cases, he said that a patient with terminal lung cancer such as Mr. Strasser, was definitely going to die in the very short term anyway, but that situations such as Mrs. Lanser's were much more complicated. Patients with emphysema could theoretically live on for a while, and doctors were often unsure whether they had done everything possible to improve their condition, even if this involved only providing short-term relief.

Contrary to Gerrit, Dr. Schuyt did not interpret the actions leading to Mr. Strasser's death as euthanasia. When I asked him whether the increased morphine had been intended to hasten Mr. Strasser's death, Dr. Schuyt answered, "In that phase of the illness it was intended to . . . alleviate suffering. Because you could see that every movement, everything, was painful. . . . But when you do that you know that death will also be hastened: that's inevitable. But it's only a question of days, maybe a week or a week and a half at most, given the rapid progression of the disease. . . . And that's not euthanasia."

He also explained his reason for not considering this to be euthanasia: "There are a lot of patients in our practice with progressive lung emphysema, with a very poor lung function, and when that deteriorates further, their condition is at least as bad as Mr. Strasser's was. It can go on for a year, five years even. And if one of those patients says that he's had enough and doesn't want to go on, and you intervene, then *that* would be euthanasia. That's a different situation to Mr. Strasser, who was clearly in the very final stage of his illness."

Although Dr. Schuyt did not consider the actions leading to the death of Mr. Strasser to be euthanasia (or Mr. Strasser's request not to suffer any longer as a euthanasia request), he did agree with Gerrit that they should increase the pain medication as a result of his request (something they would not have done in the absence of that request). Why did Dr. Schuyt agree to this increase? He may have agreed partly because the actions entailed fell outside his definition of euthanasia—for him, it was merely the continuation of the palliative treatment regimen—and partly because Mr. Strasser had terminal cancer and would certainly die within the next few days anyway. If Mr. Strasser had been suffering just as much but had a reasonable chance of living for a number of months, then Dr. Schuyt would not have acted in the same way.

Various subjective factors and personal characteristics influenced the actions, interpretations, and decisions of the doctors. These will help to explain the differences just described. In the interest of brevity, I will continue to limit the discussion to the same three doctors.

Dr. Glas sometimes spent hours with a patient during his out-patient clinic, allowing his morning clinic to extend into his afternoon clinic. Dr. Schuyt was usually capable of limiting his consultations to the official twenty minutes, always finishing his clinic more or less on time. Dr. Glas visited patients at home, outside working hours; Dr. Schuyt, as far as I know, did not. Dr. Schuyt was concise, simple, and didactic in his explanations; Dr. Glas elaborated and digressed during extended explanations, in which a simple announcement about a prognosis could develop into a philosophical exposition on the meaning of life.

The differences between Drs. Glas and Schuyt can be viewed in terms of their ability to delimit different domains. Dr. Schuyt was more inclined to separate various activities in time and space: interaction with patients was limited to clinic hours and rounds on the ward, and always within the walls of the hospital; his private life at home was completely separate from his patients and his work; his explanations were concise and to the point. For Dr. Glas, the boundaries were less clear: work gradually merged with free time, and hospital activities spilled over into the domestic space; patients had all the time they needed to say what they needed to say, and Dr. Glas took the time to expound his own views.

These remarks do not imply value judgments—both doctors did their work well, and they were equally popular with their patients—but they provide background characteristics that help us to situate and understand their different *styles* of coping with euthanasia requests.

In this discussion, I have limited myself largely to Drs. Glas and Schuyt because they are so similar in many respects (age, specialization) but can conveniently be contrasted in others. This is intended to epitomize personal differences which are much more complex in practice and which have emerged in more detail and with greater nuance in the case studies in previous chapters.

With regard to the characteristics just described, Dr. Knol takes an intermediate position, but his freedom of action was limited by the fact that he was a junior doctor who, while on the pulmonology unit, had to deal with both doctors' patients. As a result, he also had to adjust his interpretations and actions depending on which of the two specialists was ultimately responsible for the patient in question.

The ability to delimit different domains was also illustrated in the way in which euthanasia was defined and distinguished from death hastened by increasing symptom alleviation. For Dr. Glas, the line between the two was not clearly defined and shifted from one case to another. Although everyone else referred to his actions in the case of Mrs. Van Nelle as euthanasia, he defined them only as symptom alleviation. A year earlier, however, he had granted the request of an ALS patient to stop all treatment and turn off the respirator—which was the patient's right and could in no way be construed as euthanasia—and then reported it to the public prosecutor as euthanasia. Dr. Glas did not consider the distinction between euthanasia and symptom alleviation relevant: for him, the patient's experience of suffering was central, and it was this which determined his actions. As a result, he was not inclined to consider the hastening of death as a result of increased pain medication to be euthanasia, no matter how long the patient might still have lived otherwise. For Dr. Schuyt, the line between euthanasia and symptom alleviation was relatively clear and fixed: it was determined by the life expectancy of the patient. That is why he did not consider the actions that hastened the death of Mr. Strasser to be euthanasia but would have called Dr. Glas's actions in the case of Mrs. Van Nelle euthanasia. Dr. Knol had a broad definition of euthanasia: he tended to define as euthanasia all kinds of life-shortening actions that others would have called symptom alleviation (such as in the death of Mr. Strasser). He shared Dr. Schuyt's criterion of the life expectancy of the patient, but, for him, this served to distinguish justified from unjustified euthanasia rather than to distinguish euthanasia from normal medical practice. This explains why Dr. Knol agreed with (what he called) euthanasia in Mr. Strasser's case but not in the case of Mrs. Lanser.

These personal differences also influenced the way in which doctors dealt with euthanasia requests. Dr. Glas and Dr. Knol "heard" such requests sooner than Dr. Schuyt and were more inclined to discuss them with the patient. Dr. Glas was more inclined than Drs. Schuyt and Knol to grant such requests. This was further facilitated by his broader definition of palliative care: actions that Dr. Schuyt and Dr. Knol defined as euthanasia and refused to carry out as a result were interpreted as mere symptom alleviation by Dr. Glas, hence his greater inclination to carry them out. Although Dr. Schuyt would never refuse a euthanasia request he perceived as justified, he was much more reserved in his interpretation of what counted as a justified request.

Dr. Glas and Dr. Knol were more receptive to patients' euthanasia requests than Dr. Schuyt; Dr. Schuyt and Dr. Knol were more reserved when it came to granting euthanasia requests. Each doctor had an *individual style* that influenced his interpretation of, and reaction to, his patient's euthanasia requests. These styles should not be interpreted as the sole and direct causes of specific decisions or actions, but as important contributing factors that interacted with the personalities of, and relationships between, the other actors—patient, relatives, nurses—as well as with the specific context of the ward (discussed in a later section).

THE NURSES

Sometimes patients voiced a clear and consistent desire for euthanasia when talking to the nurses but then expressed doubt when questioned by a doctor. On the other hand, a patient sometimes had a clear and consistent request when dealing with doctors but expressed doubt in the presence of nurses. Also, the way in which the nurses interpreted a patient's request and the extent to which they succeeded in communicating this to the doctor, in turn, influenced the doctor's interpretation. But because the communication between doctors and nurses was often not optimal, this could also cause misunderstanding. I have already discussed different discourses, and this is particularly applicable to the communication between patient and doctor, on the one hand, and patient and nurse on the other. I usually encountered euthanasia requests in the nursing records much earlier than in the doctors' case notes. Here, I am not claiming that patients always made their euthanasia requests to nurses first. Patients sometimes broached the subject with the specialist during an outpatient clinic visit, months or even years prior to their final admittance to the hospital, at the moment when their condition was first diagnosed.

Often, the request made to the nurses was of a different nature from the one made to the doctor, even though it might have been worded similarly, because, for example, the patient knows that the doctor, not the nurses, can grant and carry out this request. A patient could easily tell a nurse, "I want a jab right now," knowing full well that the nurse was not qualified to administer a fatal "jab," with the intention of simply calling attention to his or her plight. The patient might hesitate to make the same demand of the doctor, fearing that the doctor might grant his or her request (Mrs. Jonas, for example). On the other hand, if the patient has discussed euthanasia with the doctor and the two have come to an agreement, then the patient might express doubts to the nurses that he or she wouldn't express to the doctor, for fear that the doctor might renege on his promise (Mrs. Kees, for example).

The nurses, as a group, were involved with the patients twenty-four hours a day, often quite intimately, washing them, feeding them, and comforting them in moments of emotional and physical crisis. The doctors, on the other hand, saw patients much less frequently: the junior doctors saw them once a day during rounds, the specialists, even less frequently, during weekly rounds and occasionally during outpatient clinic visits. As a result, the nurses sometimes had relevant information about the patient of which the doctor was unaware (see The 1997).

On the other hand, however, the doctor might have known the patient much longer, sometimes for years, from his outpatient clinic. He might have visited the patient at home and known the family situation intimately, as Dr. Glas did some of his patients. It is not so much a question of one party knowing the patient better but rather of each knowing the patient differently, having different kinds of information, and understanding different aspects of the patient's situation. These different sources of information, these different interpretations, then often did not complement each other because the channels of communication between doctor and nurses, particularly regarding euthanasia, were not optimal.

In the case of Mrs. Van Nelle, I continually encountered comments in the nursing report about the patient's desire for euthanasia and references to planned euthanasia discussions with Dr. Glas. Dr. Glas, however, never spoke of euthanasia in relation to Mrs. Van Nelle and, indeed, quite explicitly said that he considered his actions relating to her to be nothing more than symptom alleviation. Clearly, the doctor and nurses held different opinions about what was happening.

At one point, Dr. Glas had arranged to meet Mrs. Van Nelle, her husband, and her daughter to discuss what was to be done. In the nursing report, I read that there would be a discussion between Mrs. Van Nelle and Dr. Glas "about euthanasia." At the appointed hour, two of the nurses waited on the ward for Dr. Glas so that they could be present at the meeting. Dr. Glas arrived on the ward in a hurry and went straight to Mrs. Van Nelle's room, followed by me. When the nurses heard that Dr. Glas had already arrived, they hurried to Mrs. Van Nelle's room, only to find the door closed. They did not enter. This episode caused much resentment and was described in a paper, written by one of the nurses concerned, to illustrate the way in which doctors ignore nurses when it comes to euthanasia.

As far as I know, Dr. Glas was never aware that he had "excluded" the nurses from the discussion with Mrs. Van Nelle. Perhaps he should have enquired whether any of the nurses involved with Mrs. Van Nelle wanted to accompany him, instead of simply going straight to her room, but, on the other hand, the nurses themselves could have been slightly more assertive and knocked on the door. I was present, after all, and not because Dr. Glas always invited me to follow him wherever he went, but because I knew that the meeting was to take place and I was waiting for him. I had installed myself strategically so that it was impossible for Dr. Glas to enter Mrs. Van Nelle's room without my spotting him. The nurses could have done the same, they could have entered the room after the door had been shut, or, at least, they could have raised the matter with Dr. Glas afterward. That they did none of these was undoubt-edly related to the hierarchical relationship between doctors and nurses and, perhaps even more, to the fact that the nurses in ques-tion were relatively young and inexperienced. Whatever the case, incidents such as this were not exceptional, and they characterized the poor communication between doctors and nurses.

When the doctor's actions fell in the gray area between euthanasia and symptom alleviation, he may have failed to make clear whether the increased morphine was intended primarily to alleviate symp-toms or whether he also consciously intended to shorten the patient's life as well (for example, the cases of Mrs. Van Nelle and Mrs. Lanser). It was difficult for the nurses to distinguish between these intertwined and often implicit intentions (indeed, in such cases, doctors themselves were often not all that clear on what their own primary intention was). This led to confusion because the nurses, who were charged with actually administering the morphine, were not sure whether they were assisting in carrying out euthanasia or simply alleviating symptoms.

If arrangements for euthanasia have been made between the doc-tor and the patient in the outpatient clinic and the patient is admitted to the ward for the implementation, this can also cause consterna-tion among the nurses. They may be dissatisfied at not being in-volved in the decision-making process, and not having experienced the patient's suffering, they may not empathize with his or her request (see also, The 1997).

The relative absence of the nursing staff in this study is, in itself, a symptom of the limited communication between doctors and nurses in the hospital. Doctors (in particular the consultant specialists) and nurses had their own tasks and responsibilities, and their own geo-graphical domains in the hospital (consulting room, office, coffee room, specific tables in the cafeteria). They worked alongside each other rather than together. In routine medical situations in which a division of labor is essential, this is not necessarily a problem, but it can have consequences in social situations, such as coffee breaks or informal chat in the corridor, situations in which the euthanasia requests of patients are often discussed. The nurses often discussed patients' euthanasia requests in their coffee room during break; the doctors consulted with one another about such requests in the corridor, during lunch, or through sometimes cryptic messages in the patients' case notes.

The internal hospital hierarchy also did not facilitate communication. As Dr. Glas remarked, "Sometimes the communication isn't as good as it should be. And you also act defensively. It's easier to talk to a colleague or a junior doctor than to venture into the nurses' coffee lounge. That's something you only do sporadically." Indeed, during almost two years of research, I hardly ever saw a consultant in the nurses' coffee room, and only infrequently did I see doctors and nurses chatting informally in the corridor or the cafeteria.

The problem here is not so much that the doctors consciously ignored the nurses' opinion or found it irrelevant, but that the daily work routine, the division of labor, the separate social domains, the changing shifts in which both doctors and nurses work, the circulation of junior doctors between units, and the tremendous workload impeded adequate communication about patients' euthanasia requests. The hierarchical culture of the hospital was epitomized by lunch in the cafeteria: the odd exception notwithstanding, the consultants sat together, the junior doctors sat together, the nurses sat together, and the administrative staff sat together. If I joined Dr. Glas for lunch, I sat with the consultants, and if I went with Gerrit Knol, I sat with the junior doctors. Tables dominated by nurses were avoided. This avoidance behavior was more pronounced the higher up the medical hierarchy you went. Medical students often sat with nurses, junior doctors sometimes, and consultants almost never (Dr. Nieuwenhuis was a notable exception).

THE CULTURE OF THE WARD

How a patient's euthanasia request was received depended on, among other things, which unit he or she happened to be in. Each unit had its own culture, its own shared mentality and customs, formed by a combination of various factors, such as the kinds of diseases and types of patients treated and the personalities of the doctors and nurses. Generally, the staff on a unit had worked together over an extended period and knew one another's quirks and had developed mutual expectations and on more or less stable relationships and ways of doing things.

In gastroenterology, for example, Dr. Nieuwenhuis always held prerounds consultations with the ward doctor and the head nurse (Dr. Nieuwenhuis was a social democrat, and it was essential that all groups were represented democratically). In the AIDS unit, on the other hand, Dr. Edelman held court with only the ward doctor, and any other specialist-in-training who might happen to be attached to his unit at the time (I was also tolerated). These meetings, which resembled high-level academic teaching sessions rather than the prerounds practical discussions in gastroenterology, often lasted for hours, as a result of which Dr. Edelman sometimes had insufficient time to actually participate in the rounds himself, much to the irritation of some of the patients and nurses. The pulmonologists were always in a hurry, inevitably started rounds late, sometimes just as the nursing day shift was about to switch to the night shift, and often had no time for prerounds discussions. They did these during rounds, discussing the patients in whispers in the corridor before going in to see them.

Among the units, there were also differences in the nature of communication with the patients. This was partly related to the personalities of the doctors involved and partly to the nature of the diseases being treated. In intensive care, patients were usually too sick to communicate adequately. In addition, the large number of specialists from different disciplines who were involved in the treatment of the average intensive care patient further inhibited direct communication with the patient. In intensive care, and on the general internal ward, which had a relatively old population, there was a lot of practical work: washing patients, making beds, dressing wounds. As a result, little time was left for the discussion of questions of life and death. On other wards, such as AIDS and pulmonology, patients tended to be more active and independent, providing more opportunity for the development of euthanasia requests and for the patients to discuss these requests with the nurses.

In some units, the general consensus was that euthanasia had become a normal part of terminal care. This does not mean that it had become routine or daily practice, but that it was open for discussion; requests were not considered abnormal or a sign of mental instability on the part of the patient or a reflection of inadequate care. It meant that, under specific circumstances, a request could be honored. In other units, euthanasia could not even be discussed.

LANGUAGE, DISCOURSE, AND COMMUNICATION

To fully understand the decision-making process relating to euthanasia, it is important to study the personalities and idiosyncrasies of the various participants and the social context in which they act. It is also important to see these processes as language phenomena: a euthanasia request, a doctor's discussion of that request with colleagues, and the final decision to grant the request are all expressed through language. The interpretations that determine the decision to grant a request (was it a real request, or was the patient trying to express something else?) are based largely on verbal communication. And, if the patient dies with the physician's assistance, it is through language that those actions are interpreted and defined as euthanasia or normal medical practice.

Here, the concept of discourse is important. By discourse, I mean, simply, a more or less clearly defined and internally consistent collection of statements (which can be both spoken and written) or a more or less coherent way of speaking about a topic, or group of related topics, together with its underlying assumptions. In practice, it is possible to distinguish different discourses relating to the same phenomenon. These discourses may differ from one individual to another (two doctors, for example) or between groups (doctors and nurses or doctors and relatives).

In addition, one individual may use different, even contradictory, discourses relating to the same phenomenon. These discourses may exist separately but simultaneously (for example, when a patient repeatedly, explicitly, and consistently tells the nurses that he or she wants euthanasia but is not really ready when talking to the doctor), or they may be intertwined and difficult to distinguish (as when a patient continually expresses an explicit and consistent request for euthanasia, while sending out implicit and equally consistent signals that he or she does not want to die).

In practice, there are usually multiple, sometimes contradictory interpretations with regard to a patient and his or her euthanasia request. This indeterminacy also applies to retrospective interpretations after the patient has died.

Mrs. Kees expressed a consistent desire for euthanasia when talking to the attending physician, Dr. Hansen, and she confirmed this in an interview with Dr. Nieuwenhuis as part of the official euthanasia procedure. However, when she talked to the nurses, she allowed doubts to show through. "When she talks to me her request is consistent," Mark Hansen told me, "but when she talks to the nurses sometimes she says things like 'Well, I'm not in pain right now, and I can still see the children, so I can for a while still hold out . . . .' But then when I come along, or the internist, then she really wants it to go ahead on Wednesday [the day on which euthanasia had been planned]."

When Inge Fransen, the head nurse, visited her, Mrs. Kees said, "It's already Monday, not long to Wednesday now." Inge interpreted this as doubt and asked her whether she had second thoughts. "On the one hand, I do," Mrs. Kees answered, "because I want to live, though only if I can be healthy. But whether it happens today or tomorrow, I'm going to die anyway, so then it's better to do it my way." In the medical report someone had written, "She says that she wants to go ahead, but she has told the nurses that she can always change her mind if she wants to." Underneath, Mieke van der Ven, the anesthetist, had written, "Does she want to or doesn't she?"

Here, two discourses can be distinguished: a consistent, explicit, and adamant one, expressed to Mark Hansen, who, as the patient's doctor, was responsible for actually carrying out the euthanasia, and Dr. Nieuwenhuis, who had to officially support Mark's decision, and a more uncertain and implicit one when talking to the nurses. In her interactions with the anesthetist, who was also involved in carrying out the euthanasia, there was a certain amount of overlap: she expressed doubt but, at the same time, insisted that the appointment be kept. If she had expressed doubt to Mark Hansen or Dr. Nieuwenhuis, then the euthanasia probably would have been delayed or canceled, which she did not want. She did, however, apparently experience a need to express certain feelings that might be interpreted either as doubt and hesitation or as an expression of the reluctance with which she approached her inevitable death. She aired these latter sentiments to the nurses and, to a lesser extent, to the anesthetist. It is possible that she did this consciously because she knew this would not affect the decision to grant her request.

When Dr. Glas decided to increase Mrs. Van Nelle's morphine, she said that she was glad that he was finally going to deliver her from her suffering, and she refused physiotherapy, saying that it was unnecessary because she wasn't "going to be around much longer anyway." However, just after the anesthetist inserted the intravenous line, but before Dr. Glas actually connected the morphine, Mrs. Van Nelle borrowed three books from the hospital library. This did not give the impression that she knew she was going to die that same evening. Then, when Dr. Glas came to start the morphine, she complained that it was all happening "rather quickly." It was decided that Dr. Glas would wait until she went to bed, but she skipped her usual afternoon nap. In the evening she told Dr. Glas that she would only allow him to give her morphine if he could guarantee that it would not make her drowsy (even though she knew that this was impossible). After the morphine had been started and stopped several times during the course of the evening, it was finally started again, at Mrs. Van Nelle's request, just before midnight, and the next morning she was dead.

Mrs. Van Nelle used an explicit discourse in which she continually demanded euthanasia from almost everyone she encountered, while simultaneously sending out clear signals that she did not want to die. The contrast between these two discourses became very clear in the final phase.

In the case of Mr. Joost, the definition of the "natural" situation shifted continually, and Mrs. Joost implicitly accepted these shifts. Unaware that the nasogastric feeding had been stopped, she asked one of the nurses whether her husband was still being fed. When the nurse answered that he was not, Mrs. Joost simply said, "Oh," and walked away. She canceled an appointment that the internist had made with her to explain why they had stopped feeding her husband, saying that she had to go somewhere and did not *really* need to see the doctor. It was clear what had been agreed, she said. She gave the impression that she knew exactly what was going on but did not want to be explicitly informed about everything, or to make the major decisions herself. At the same time, however, she knew quite well in which direction things were moving, and by strategically refusing to say anything explicitly, she made the decisions nonetheless, clearly indicating how far the doctors were permitted to go.

"Sooner or later we'll have to think about what we're going to do," Mark Hansen had said during his first meeting with Mrs. Joost. "For example, if he gets pneumonia, then we could treat the pain and shortness of breath, but not the primary infection." Mrs. Joost interrupted Mark to indicate that she didn't want active euthanasia, but she agreed with the symptom alleviation. Mark interpreted this as a sign that Mr. Joost's relatives were against active euthanasia but in favor of abstinence/passive euthanasia. This meant that they would not treat Mr. Joost if he developed complications. Mark's interpretation was later confirmed by Mrs. Joost.

Mrs. Joost was capable of switching to a very explicit discourse if she felt that her implicit messages were being interpreted wrongly or her wishes ignored, for example, when she realized that the internist and the anesthetist had given her husband antibiotics to counter a nascent pneumonia.

A narrow definition of euthanasia, combined with a largely implicit discourse, made it possible for Mrs. Joost (who was a Catholic) to allow (and even order) the gradual reduction of life-prolonging interventions without moral dilemma. She could make clear that she agreed with the termination of certain interventions without actually saying so.

I have been discussing discrete but internally relatively consistent discourses. However, the euthanasia requests of many patients were embedded in discourses that were anything but consistent. Sometimes the manner in which the request surfaced was related to the patient's illness trajectory, and sometimes it was related to the patient's emotional state. A euthanasia request, even one that is explicit and consistent, may also serve to express things other than just the desire to terminate life, and it requires substantial interpretative skills on the part of the physician to make the right decision, especially if the patient employs different discourses in communication with his or her family, the doctors, the nurses, and the psychologist. In such cases, there may not be a single "correct" interpretation, and multiple, even contradictory interpretations of the same situation are possible.

This is further complicated by the fact that, in practice, the word *euthanasia* is not always used unequivocally, and actions that are officially defined as euthanasia cannot always be conveniently distinguished from other actions that hasten the end of life but are not euthanasia. In practice, what counts as euthanasia is socially and culturally constructed in specific contexts. This will be discussed in the next chapter.

Chapter 12

What Is Euthanasia?

In the Dutch literature, medical actions that hasten the end of life have been classified in a variety of ways, and different definitions have come and gone during the past twenty years. More recently, a consensus has developed, and the definition used by the State Committee on Euthanasia in its 1985 report is now generally accepted as the "official" definition: "Euthanasia is the deliberate termination of a person's life by another person at the former's request." The distinction between active and passive euthanasia and the concept of involuntary euthanasia are no longer part of the Dutch discussion. This narrowing of definitions in the formal discussion is not reflected in the way the term is used in practice, and many of those involved employ their own, often idiosyncratic definitions, which may also vary from one situation to another.

In theory, at least, there appears to be no compelling reason (and certainly not from an etymological viewpoint—euthanasia means good death) why the term *euthanasia* should be limited to "the deliberate termination of a person's life by another person at the former's request." This restriction stems from the desire to develop a legal framework for the regulation of euthanasia in the Netherlands. Indeed, three of the major studies of euthanasia that have been published in the Netherlands during the 1990s have all been motivated by the quest for just such a legal framework (Van der Maas, van Delden, and Pijnenborg 1991; Van der Wal 1992; Van der Wal and Van der Maas 1996).

The State Commission definition is concise and clear enough to form the basis for legal regulation (all the messy, ambiguous situations involving an increase in pain medication, accompanied by equivocal intentions on the part of the physician, are avoided), and, perhaps more significantly, it fits perfectly with Article 293 of the Dutch Penal Code: He who takes the life of another at the latter's explicit and serious request will be punished with a prison term not exceeding twelve years.

Although an unambiguous and generally accepted definition of euthanasia is, in many respects, desirable, particularly with regard to (legal) control, it can also lead to problems, if it is interpreted as a reflection of clinical practice. In practice, various, often vague and implicit definitions of euthanasia are used, and the line between euthanasia and other actions that hasten the end of life cannot be clearly drawn.

EUTHANASIA AND ASSISTED SUICIDE

It has become clear from my research that, in practice, doctors and patients frequently refer to various actions that hasten the end of life as euthanasia, though they are not euthanasia according to the "official" definition. This applies particularly to assisted suicide. For example, in the negotiations that led up to David's death (see Chapter 1) and in all the interviews and discussions about his request, those involved only spoke about euthanasia. I never once heard anyone mention suicide or assisted suicide, and I never encountered these terms in the written reports and comments in the medical records, describing cases in which patients had taken a euthanaticum supplied by the doctor. Dr. Edelman made agreements with David and Bryan about *euthanasia*, and he left it up to them to decide whether they wanted to die quickly or slowly, and whether they wanted to take the euthanaticum themselves or have him administer it. In other words, the difference between taking the euthanaticum yourself and having it administered by the doctor was, for those involved, of the same order as the difference between the fast and the slow method; that is, it was a technical distinction related to the way in which euthanasia was carried out rather than a qualitative difference between two different kinds of action.

Whether a particular case of hastening the end of life turns out to be euthanasia or assisted suicide is often dependent on arbitrary circumstances. In the case of Mrs. Kees, it was the nausea caused by the tumor in her stomach that prevented her from taking the euthanaticum herself, as she had originally intended. With Bryan Mayflower, it was his life insurance policy that determined his choice.

The boundary between euthanasia and assisted suicide is not always clear. If a doctor and a patient have agreed on assisted suicide, but the doctor holds the cup to the patient's mouth because the patient is too weak to lift it, is that still assisted suicide, or is it euthanasia? Does the difference lie in the lifting of the cup or in the act of swallowing? In the case of assisted suicide, patients usually self-administer the euthanaticum orally. But, as Van der Wal has pointed out, the doctor could also administer the euthanaticum orally. Van der Wal further speculates about whether it is the means of administering or the person who administers that determines the difference. What about cases in which the doctor intervenes when the patient threatens to recover after self-administering the euthanaticum (Van der Wal 1992:99)?

If we speculate further and assume that Bryan Mayflower died because he himself radically increased the flow of morphine through the pump with the intention of killing himself, would that be suicide, or would it be assisted suicide because Dr. Edelman allowed Bryan to administer his own pain medication, while also drawing his attention to the fact that an increase might be fatal? Or perhaps we should call it euthanasia because he would have increased the morphine under the direct responsibility of Dr. Edelman, just as it would have been euthanasia if Dr. Edelman had instructed an assistant to administer the fatal dose? Or does it all depend on the intentions of those involved? More recently, an attempt has been made to delineate the boundaries more clearly by defining various borderline cases in which the doctor actively intervenes as euthanasia, but the basic problem remains (Van der Wal and Van der Maas 1996).

In 1991, the Remmelink Commission concluded that the difference between euthanasia and assisted suicide was simply one of the technical means of execution, seeing that the participants have the same aim in both cases. The commission concluded further that the distinction between euthanasia and assisted suicide was not relevant for its discussion of the nature and context of actions that hasten the end of life (Van der Maas, van Delden, and Pijnenborg 1991:13).

I have always wondered why this distinction is made at all. In the Netherlands, it probably stems from the fact that the penal code distinguishes between the two (in Articles 293 and 294). In the United States and other countries, the emphasis on physician-assisted suicide rather than euthanasia probably serves to emphasize the free will of the patient in the face of formidable opposition to euthanasia and fear of the "slippery slope." In the Netherlands, evidence suggests that physicians prefer assisted suicide to euthanasia. In 1995, the executive committee of the Royal Dutch Medical Association (KNMG) expressed a preference for assisted suicide because this optimized the patient's right of self-determination (Legemate 1998:27).

If the generally accepted definition of euthanasia entails a conscious and well-considered request by the patient, then the distinction between euthanasia and assisted suicide is rather artificial. The important factor here is that, in both cases, the individual decides that he or she no longer wants to live, and this person then involves a doctor to assist with the technical aspects of realizing this wish. If we need to use a single term for these actions, then assisted suicide would seem more appropriate, if the emphasis is to be on the locus of the decision and the fact that another person is involved in carrying it out. If the emphasis is to be on the fact that it is a "good death" which is being sought, then euthanasia would be the more appropriate term for both kinds of action. Indeed, in publications, as in clinical practice generally, the term euthanasia is used for the sake of convenience to refer to both actions.

EUTHANASIA AND SYMPTOM ALLEVIATION

In the distinction between euthanasia and assisted suicide, the intention of those involved is the same but the technical means of carrying it out differs; in the distinction between euthanasia and death as a result of increasing pain medication, this is the other way round: the technical execution can be exactly the same, and the difference lies in the intentions of those involved.

According to a recent study, the number of cases of increased pain medication and/or symptom alleviation in which the doctor took into account the probability or the certainty that the patient's death would thereby be hastened was estimated to be 19.1 percent of all deaths in the Netherlands in 1995. In 2.9 percent of these deaths, the hastening of the patient's death was also partly intended (Van der Wal and Van der Maas 1996:77, 92).

My research has shown that it is extremely difficult to establish what "taking into account the probability or the certainty that the patient's death would thereby be hastened" and "the partly intended hastening of the patient's death" mean. When a doctor is confronted with the choice between these and various other options on a questionnaire, he or she might not have much difficulty in choosing an answer, but such answers do not give us much insight into the subtleties and ambiguities of real-life situations. Complex situations, motives, and decisions become simpler and more consistent when they are reconstructed afterward. People continually restructure and reorder their memories, partly because of the influence of new experiences and partly to economize. So when you question a doctor about the reasons for a particular decision months after it was made, then he or she is likely to tell you the motives that are foremost in his or her mind at present, motives that may already be the product of several interpretations.

Although it has been largely ignored in various major studies, the so-called "gray area" between euthanasia and symptom alleviation is extremely important for the discussion about euthanasia. Exactly the same equipment, substances, and way of administering them can be used for symptom alleviation *and* euthanasia, and given that a patient might request euthanasia *and* medically require a considerable increase in pain medication, it is only the physician's own interpretation of his or her motive that determines whether his or her actions are euthanasia or normal medical practice. In situations such as this, a patient requests euthanasia and the doctor grants that request, without intending to, but knowing quite well that he or she cannot do otherwise.

The situation becomes more complicated when the doctor's intentions are equivocal (for example, the doctor is not sure whether he or she wants to grant the patient's request), or when the doctor has decided to grant the patient's request at a later date and a sudden increase in the patient's experience of pain necessitates increasing the morphine, as a result of which the patient dies. In cases such as these, the actions that grant the patient's request for euthanasia are simultaneously the only actions that are medically and ethically acceptable, given the patient's pain.

These are not simply hypothetical cases. In the case of Mr. Strasser, for example, his request was "not to suffer any longer." It was possible to interpret this request in two ways: as a request for euthanasia or simply as a request not to suffer any longer (although the fact that he then proceeded to say good-bye to everybody seems to suggest that he interpreted it as the former). This is how Gerrit Knol, the ward doctor, interpreted it, and when he increased the morphine, it was with the intention of granting a euthanasia request. However, Dr. Schuyt, the consultant who was ultimately responsible and under whose responsibility the morphine was administered, interpreted Mr. Strasser's request simply as a desire not to suffer unnecessary pain, and when he gave instructions to increase the morphine, it was solely with that intention in mind.

But was that "really" his intention, or did he just interpret it that way (for me and for himself) because it was more convenient and because he had no other option anyway? His interpretation was probably influenced by his definition of euthanasia, as he had frequently explained it to me: that if a patient was in the final stages of illness, and had only a few hours or days at most to live, and was in pain, then a lethal increase in the morphine dosage was not euthanasia. Here, the physician's "intention" is partly determined by his definition of euthanasia.

The causes of pain cannot always be objectively established, and it is possible that a person may suffer excruciating pain in the absence of any clear physical basis and in spite of large doses of morphine (as occurred with Mrs. Van Nelle and Bryan Mayflower). It is therefore possible that a doctor can only free a patient from pain by killing him or her with a massive increase in the morphine dosage. In the case of Mr. Oosten, it was, according to Albert Meertens, the patient's shortness of breath that kept him breathing. Relieving his shortness of breath and killing him were one and the same action.

EUTHANASIA AND THE WITHDRAWAL OR NONIMPLEMENTATION OF LIFE-PROLONGING TREATMENT

The ambiguities discussed previously also apply to the distinction between euthanasia and the withdrawal or nonimplementation of life-prolonging treatment. A patient may submit a request for euthanasia that the doctor considers legitimate, but instead of administering a euthanaticum, he withdraws life-prolonging treatment (turns off the respirator, for example) or gives instructions not to reanimate, even though he expects a cardiac arrest. Just as in the case of death due to an increase in pain medication, these actions all fall in the category of "normal medical practice." Here, however, the *intentions* of those involved play no role. This is strange because the intention is quite clearly to allow the patient to die.

The withdrawal of a life-prolonging treatment is an active and deliberate action. Take the case of Mr. Joost, for example. The specialists initially attempted to wean him from the respirator, and they tried to arrange a place for him in a special nursing home. When it became clear that Mr. Joost could not survive without the respirator and that the nursing home had such a long waiting list that he would certainly be dead before a vacancy arose, the doctors decided to abstain from treating complications, and, as a result, Mr. Joost eventually died. The withholding of life-prolonging therapy and the decision not to treat opportunistic infections were part of a passive policy of abstinence. However, the withdrawal of artificial feeding, fluids, and nonpalliative medicine and the gradual phasing out of the respirator can only be interpreted as active interventions intended to hasten Mr. Joost's death.

Mrs. Lanser said that she wanted to die. Gerrit Knol noted this in her medical report as a request for euthanasia. Dr. Glas said that he supported her wish, but he did not interpret it as a euthanasia request. Rather, he saw it as a request for the withdrawal of life-prolonging therapy. He therefore gave instructions to stop all nonpalliative medicines, he increased the amount of oxygen she was receiving, and he increased the dose of morphine to relieve her shortness of breath. If we ignore the complications caused by the disagreements among the relatives, for the moment, then it is clear that the patient's request, the doctor's endorsement, and the sequence of actions that led to the patient's death could just as easily have been classified as euthanasia or the withdrawal of life-prolonging therapy, the only difference being the interpretation that Dr. Glas himself made of his own actions.

This is also clear in the case of Mr. Strasser, which Gerrit Knol interpreted as euthanasia and Dr. Schuyt as palliative abstinence (*palliatief abstinerend beleid*) and, therefore, not euthanasia.

EUTHANASIA AS CULTURAL CONSTRUCT

In the public discussion about euthanasia in the Netherlands, it is often assumed that all care providers utilize the same official definition of euthanasia, that decision-making situations at the end of life are unambiguous, that motives and intentions can be unequivocally interpreted and objectively described, that subjective factors do not play a significant role, and that there is a single determinate discourse through which doctors and patients communicate. This book has sought to show that these assumptions are mistaken.

The way in which euthanasia is defined officially appears to be clear, concise, and practical, but, in fact, euthanasia is thereby *constructed* as a separate category: one aspect of a continuous practice is marked out and made the object of legal control and possible sanctions. However, because various types of life-shortening action by physicians are continuous in practice, it is often possible for those involved to adjust their definitions and their interpretations so that their actions do not fall within the scope of the official definition. They do not necessarily do this consciously, to hide cases of euthanasia or to avoid control, but unconsciously, and as a result of the ambiguities inherent in practical situations. If a situation is equivocal, then those involved are likely to choose the interpretation that is most favorable for them on pragmatic grounds.

This process of interpretation is made more complicated by the different, sometimes idiosyncratic definitions of euthanasia that various individual participants utilize. These definitions—which often are not made explicit—frequently deviate substantially from that which forms the basis for control and legislation. Moreover, in specific situations, different individual participants may have diverse opinions as to whether their actions constitute euthanasia. Also, one individual can utilize different interpretations of the same actions depending on the situation and with whom he or she is talking. Once again, this may not be conscious manipulation of the "facts," but a consequence of the indeterminacy of the actions and situations in question.

In practice, euthanasia is constructed as such in the discourse of those involved. This does not mean that any life-shortening action by a physician can be interpreted as euthanasia, or that any case of euthanasia can be made into something else by simply reinterpreting it as such. However, a whole range of life-shortening actions by physicians can be interpreted in different ways, and it is in the participants' discourse—how they speak and write about their actions—that these actions are defined as euthanasia or normal medical practice.

This has consequences for the monitoring and control of euthanasia—which is what the entire public debate in the Netherlands is basically about. In the final instance, any workable system of monitoring will have to depend on the way in which the participants—in particular, the doctors—interpret their decisions and actions, and as long as there is wide variation in this, monitoring is going to be inadequate.

Appendix

Euthanasia Declaration

NAME:_____

DATE OF BIRTH:_____

PLACE OF BIRTH:_____

After thorough consideration, by my own free will and in full possession of my faculties, I declare the following:

I. In case I, at any time, as a result of illness, accident, or any other cause, enter into a physical and/or mental state from which recovery to a reasonable and dignified state is unlikely, then I wish:

    A. that no means or techniques are applied to me with the intention of maintaining or prolonging physical life processes;

    B. that no means or techniques are applied to me with the intention of maintaining or reviving a conscious state in me;

    C. that euthanasia is carried out on me.

II. If I find myself in a state as indicated in Part I, but fully conscious, then the attending physician should obtain a confirmation of this declaration from me; in case I am mentally incapable of participating in such a consultation, then this declaration must be considered as my expressed wish.

Date: _____ Signature: _____

Notes

Preface

1. In practice, in clinical settings, the situation is less clear-cut, as the following chapters will show.

2. For the sake of convenience I refer to both euthanasia and assisted suicide as euthanasia.

3. Using the same methodology, another anthropologist carried out a similar study among nurses in the pulmonology unit of a large university hospital (1,000 beds) in the north of the country (The 1997).

4. The number of patients suffering from each disease was as follows:

Lung cancer	25
Lung cancer and emphysema	2
Gastrointestinal cancer	5
ALS	2
AIDS	21
Total	55

Chapter 1

1. I use the term "euthanasia declaration" as a literal translation of the Dutch *euthanasieverklaring* rather than "living will" or "advance directive," as these terms (for which there are also Dutch equivalents: *levenstestament* and *niet-reanimeerverklaring*) do not refer to euthanasia. See the Appendix for a translation of the euthanasia declaration issued by the Association for Voluntary Euthanasia in the Netherlands.

2. "Ranstad Hospital" is a fictitious name.

Chapter 4

1. In Dutch, *levensbeëindiging* literally means "the termination of life." This term and the related *levensbeëindigend handelen*—"action to terminate life" are frequently used to refer to euthanasia, although they are much looser in meaning.

2. A *palliatief abstinerend beleid,* literally a "policy of palliative abstention," is a common expression in the context of treatment of terminally ill patients. It

means that the only treatment given is palliative and that any treatment that would not alleviate symptoms but only extend the patient's life is withheld.

Chapter 6

1. The order of chapters in the final version of the book changed, so the first five chapters that were written are not the same as the first five in the present book.

2. I managed to persuade participants to allow me to report everything literally. The only things that have been altered in this presentation are the names of the partcipants, the name of the hospital, and some of the dates.

3. For a critique of this, see Pool 1994:233-240.

References

Bernard, H.R., P. Killworth, D. Kronenveld, and L. Sailer (1984). The problem of informant accuracy. *Annual Review of Anthropology* 13:495-517.

Bloch, M. and J. Parry (1982). *Death and the Regeneration of Life.* Cambridge: Cambridge University Press.

Clifford, J. (1983). On ethnographic authority. *Representations* 2:132-143.

Enthoven, L. (1988). *Het Recht op Leven en Dood.* Deventer, the Netherlands: Kluwer.

Fabian, J. (1990). *Power and Performance.* Madison, WI: University of Wisconsin Press.

Freeman, L.C., A.K. Romney, and S.C. Freeman (1987). Cognitive structure and informant accuracy. *American Anthropologist* 89:310-325.

Heider, K.G. (1988). The Rashomon effect: When ethnographers disagree. *American Anthropologist* 90:73-81.

Hockey, J. (1990). *Experiences of Death: An Anthropological Account.* Edinburgh: Edinburgh University Press.

Kellehear, A. (1990). *Dying of Cancer: The Final Year of Life.* London: Harwood Academic Publishers.

Kleinman, A. (1980). *Patients and Healers in the Context of Culture.* Berkeley, CA: University of California Press.

Leenen, H.J.J. (1988). *Handboek Gezondheidsrecht: Rechten van Mensen in de Gezondheidszorg* (Tweede druk). Alphen aan den Rijn: Samsom.

Legemate, J. (1998). De juridische context van euthanasie en de inhoud van de zorgvuldigheidsregels. In J. Legemate and R.J.M. Dillman (Eds.), *Levensbeëindigend Handelen door een Arts: Tussen Norm en Praktijk.* Houten/Diegem: Bohn Stafleu Van Loghum, pp. 26-44.

Legemate, J. and R. J. M. Dillman. (1998). 25 jaar discussie over levensbeëindigend handelen door artsen. In J. Legemate. and R. J. M. Dillman (Eds.), *Levensbeëindigend Handelen door een Arts: Tussen Norm en Praktijk.* Houten/ Diegem: Bohn Stafleu Van Loghum, pp. 1-10.

Melief, W.B.A.M. (1991). *De Zorg voor Terminale Patienten en de Omgang met Euthanasie door Hulpverleners in de Thuiszorg en de Intramurale Zorg.* Den Haag: NIMAWO,

Middleton, J. (1982). Lugbara death. In M. Bloch and J. Parry (Eds.), *Death and the Regeneration of Life.* Cambridge: Cambridge University Press, pp. 134-154.

Palgi, P. and H. Abramovitch. (1984). Death: A cross-cultural perspective. *Annual Review of Anthropology* 13:385-417.

Parry, J. (1982). Sacrificial death and the necrophagous ascetic. In M. Bloch and J. Parry (Eds.), *Death and the Regeneration of Life*. Cambridge: Cambridge University Press, pp. 74-110.

Pool, R. (1992). De sociale context van beslissingen rond het levenseinde. In J. Fiselier en F. Strijbosch (Eds.), *Cultuur en Delict, Speciale Uitgave van Recht der Werkelijkheid*. Den Haag: VUGA Uitgeverij, pp. 71-82.

Pool, R. (1994). *Dialogue and the Interpretation of Illness. Conversations in a Cameroon Village*. Oxford: Berg Publishers.

Pratt, M.L. (1986). Fieldwork in common places. In J. Clifford and G. Marcus (Eds.), *Writing Culture: The Poetics and Politics of Ethnography*. Berkeley, CA: University of California Press, pp. 27-50.

Rosaldo, R. (1989). *Culture and Truth: The Remaking of Social Analysis*. Boston, MA: Beacon Press.

Saville-Troike, M. (1982). *The Ethnography of Communication*. Oxford: Blackwell.

Slomka, J. (1992). The negotiation of death: Clinical decision making at the end of life. *Social Science and Medicine* 35(3):251-259.

Tedlock, D. (1983). *The Spoken Word and the Work of Interpretation*. Philadelphia, PA: University of Pennsylvania Press.

The, A.-M. (1997). *"Vanavond om 8 uur . . ." Verpleegkundige dilemma's bij euthanasie en Andere Beslissingen Rond het Levenseinde*. Houten/Diegem: Bohn Stafleu Van Loghum.

Tyler, S. (1987). On "writing-up/off" as "speaking-for." *Journal of Anthropological Research* 43(4):338-342.

Van der Maas, P., J.J.M. Van Delden, and L. Pijnenborg (1991). *Medische Beslissingen Rond het Levenseinde. Het onderzoek voor de Commissie Onderzoek Medische Praktijk inzake Euthanasie*. The Hague: SDU Uitgeverij. Published in English as Van der Maas, P.J., J.J.M. Van Delden, and L. Pijnenborg (1992). Euthanasia and other medical decisions concerning the end of life. *Health Policy* 22(1/2).

Van der Maas, P.J., G. Van der Wal, and I. Haverkate, C.L.M. de Graaf, J.G.C. Kester, D.B.D. Onwuteaka-Philipsen, A. Van der Heide, J.M. Bosma, and D.L. Willems (1996). Euthanasia, physician-assisted suicide, and other medical practices involving the end of life in the Netherlands 1990-1995. *New England Journal of Medicine* 335:1699-1705.

Van der Wal, G. (1992). *Euthanasie en Hulp bij Zelfdoding door Huisartsen*. Rotterdam, Netherlands: WYT Uitgeefgroep.

Van der Wal, G. and P.J. Van der Maas (1996). *Euthanasie en Andere Medische Beslissingen Ronde het Levenseinde. De Praktijk en de Meldingsprocedure*. The Hague: SDU Uitgevers.

Van der Wal, G., P.J. Van der Maas, and J.M. Bosma, B.D. Onwuteaka-Philipsen, D.L. Willems, A. Van der Heide, and P.J. Kostense (1996). Evaluation of the notification procedure for physician-assisted death in the Netherlands. *New England Journal of Medicine* 335:1706-1711.

Index

Printed in the United States
by Baker & Taylor Publisher Services